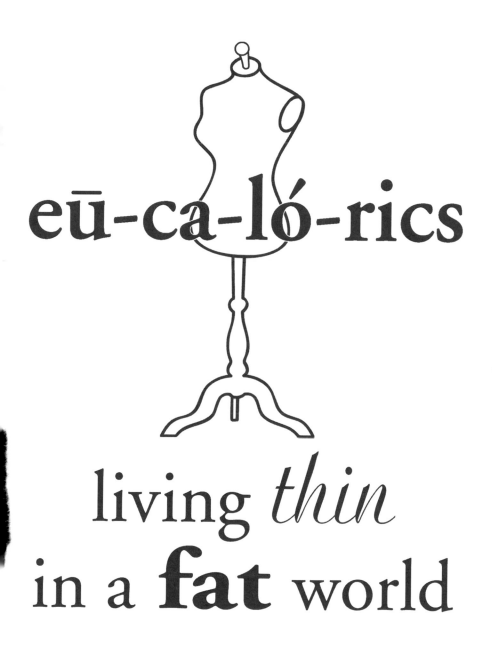

eū-ca-ló-rics

living *thin*
in a **fat** world

Jackie and Diane Scott
with Brett A. Scott, M.D.

Disclaimer

The information provided in this book is intended for reference only. This book is designed to help you make informed decisions about your health, but is no substitute for the advice and treatment that may have been prescribed to you by your doctor. Please consult your personal physician before making any changes in your diet or beginning a new exercise regime.

First Printing
January 2004

Copyright © 2003
JANDDCO, Inc.

"eū-ca-ló-rics: Living thin in a fat world" is printed by Host Communications, Inc., 904 North Broadway, Lexington, KY 40505.

ISBN: 1-57640-085-9

Acknowledgements

Special thanks to David and Jackie Bondurant, our first Eucalorics guinea pigs. The First United Methodist Church of Lexington, Ky., who allowed us to use their commercial kitchen, and the participants in the Temple Reconstruction Project who ate chef surprise night after night as we developed and perfected the recipes that appear in *Eucalorics.*

John Andrews who provided encouragement, created artwork and critiqued manuscripts.

Stephanie Peterson, Kim Troxall and Host Communications who helped transform a work in progress into a finished product.

Forward

Do you not know that your body is a temple of the Holy Spirit, who is in you,
whom you received from God? You are not your own;
1 Corinthians 6:19

I remember thinking, "Does some new diet really qualify as a ministry?" when I learned of Jackie and Diane's request to offer The Temple Reconstruction Project at our church. They were to provide nutritional counseling and prepare healthy dinners to a group of volunteer dieters. The experiences and observations that would soon follow convinced me that what they have to offer really is life changing!

The first clue came when I compared Jackie and Diane to their pictures in our church directory from just two years earlier. The difference was astonishing. What they had learned and were practicing was clearly working. Their weight loss was steady and sustained. Instead of looking unhealthy and acting lethargic, as is often the case with people who go on fad diets, they looked wonderful and full of energy.

My wife, LaVonda, had been struggling for more than ten years, since the birth of our last child, with being overweight. She was unhappy and self-conscious about her weight. I showed her our newsletter article about The Temple Reconstruction Project and suggested that she become one of the volunteers.

LaVonda got involved, and over the next eighteen months, lost sixty-five pounds. The number of pounds tells only a small part of the story. Her success was noticed and frequently complimented by our friends. I was happy to support her progress by agreeing to frequent replacements in her wardrobe as sizes got smaller. The results continue. She is obviously happier, far more confident, and full of energy. I am very proud of her.

Her diet involved changes in some of the foods that we purchase and prepare. Our whole family can comfortably live with these changes because meals taste good and portions are satisfying. She was able to commit to a very reasonable exercise plan that does not require endless sore muscles and a complete reorganization of our schedules. The change is more than just a temporary diet plan for losing weight, but it is a lifestyle change that is reasonable enough to stay committed to. The result is that her weight loss is sustained and we are all eating healthier.

Since starting The Temple Reconstruction Project, Jackie and Diane have been volunteering their time and expertise as our church's resident chefs.

Their enthusiasm and great care in serving great tasting, healthier foods has earned them the opportunity to challenge, coach and engage all of our folks with their...well, ministry! They have offered us so much in our efforts to live with joy and freedom and to be great stewards of the gift of our health.

I am very proud and honored to recommend *eū-ca-ló-rics: Living Thin in a Fat World* , as I believe that Jackie and Diane have filled it with the same energy, enthusiasm, proven advice, and genuine care with which they continue serving us so wonderfully. Blessings and Bon Appetit!

Rev. Ken Klemme
Pastor of Outreach & Evangelism
First United Methodist Church
Lexington, Kentucky

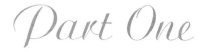

Part One

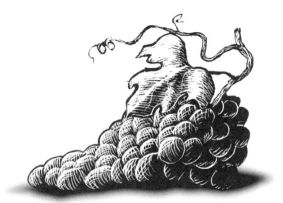

Eucalorics

chapter 1

Realistic Expectations

L osing weight is the modern day quest. The search for the famed city of El Dorado, the fountain of youth, the impossible dream. Most of us have experienced many diet failures and each failure makes it harder and harder to believe that any long-term solution exists. But we haven't given up hope. We're still looking.

When we're looking for a solution to our weight problems, what do we want? A quick fix. Advertise quick weight loss and we will buy anything. Advertise quick weight loss and we will believe everything — outrageous statements, ridiculous promises, absurd testimonials. Hook, line and sinker.

"And here's the fabulous new weight loss product you've been hearing so much about, 'Dr. Ima Lyer's Weight Loss Elixir.' Dr. Lyer, I.M.D., received her Imaginary Medical Degree from a highly respected mail order university just last month. Her extensive research has discovered a previously overlooked medical phenomenon that causes amazingly quick weight loss.

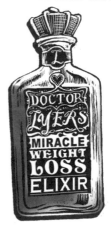

"Dr. Lyer's Weight Loss Elixir comes in handy, single-serving-sized bottles and tastes like chocolate. When consumed at bedtime, it acts as a sleeping aid, induces lovely dreams in technicolor, and dissolves fat while you sleep. But wait — that's not all, folks! It tightens skin, improves your complexion, and hardens your nails. Of course, there's no unpleasant exercise, and you can lose weight while continuing to eat anything you want. And we're practically giving it away! A one month supply for the bargain price of $19.95.

"Order within the next fifteen minutes, and we'll include an additional month's supply at no extra charge. Be one of our first 100 callers and you'll also receive a jar of our specially formulated cellulite cream, valued at $29.95, absolutely free. In addition to reducing cellulite and eliminating stretch marks, this amazing cream removes warts and prevents hair loss. Order now. Supplies are limited."

No matter how incredible the claims, we appear to be easy prey for any and all weight loss advertising. Lose 10 pounds in 48 hours! You bet, sign me up. Pills and potions that melt weight away! Sounds great, where do I send my money? Snake-oil salesmen are alive and well, and they're getting rich selling weight loss elixirs and magic beans.

How has everyone reached such levels of desperation? We're fat. And, despite spending lots of time, effort and money trying to lose weight, we keep getting fatter.

What effect have our diet failures had on our weight loss goals? Very little. Even though we're moving further and further away from those goals, we're not willing to change them. We just spend more money on magic beans.

Ambitious Goals

Ask any of us, no matter our present weight, and we all want to weigh less. A little less? No. A little less is not good enough. We want to weigh a lot less. What is it about human nature that causes us to struggle so determinedly against being average? When I was overweight, I was stunningly overweight. But when I began to diet, did I pick the average female number to strive for? Of course not.

The mythical "average female" is reported to be 5'4", a size 14 and to weigh 148 pounds. But I'm only 5'2". Since I'm shorter than the average woman, I obviously need to weigh less. Never mind that I weighed 99 pounds more than the average woman. When I decided to do something about it, suddenly average wasn't good enough. I hadn't weighed less than 200 pounds in ten years, but in my mind, weighing 148 pounds wasn't sufficient. Was I crazy? Yes. But I was not alone.

On any given day, 25 percent of the men and 40 percent of the women in this country are on a diet. Statistics from weight loss programs indicate that most people stay on a diet eight to 12 weeks and lose about 20 pounds.

These programs consider a diet successful if 10 to 15 percent of total body weight is lost. This level of weight loss can also produce statistically significant improvement in those medical conditions that are related to being overweight, such as high blood pressure and Type 2 diabetes. The typical dieter, however, sets far more lofty goals.

In a study of overweight women, whose average weight was 220 pounds, members of the group selected 135 pounds as a dream weight. This represented a 38 percent reduction in body weight. Their happy weight was 150 pounds, a 32 percent reduction in body weight; their acceptable weight was 164 pounds, a 25 percent reduction in body weight. The group indicated they would be disappointed in a 10 to 15 percent weight loss. A 10 percent loss would be 22 pounds; a 15 percent loss would be 33 pounds.

Why would anyone be disappointed in a weight loss of 33 pounds? We're not satisfied with losing weight. We want to be thin. No matter how heavy we are, we don't want to be less heavy. We want to be thin.

What else do we want?
- We want to be thin **now**.
- We want it to be easy to **get** thin.
- We want it to be easy to **stay** thin.

When it comes to losing weight, we want instantaneous, painless and permanent results.

Verbal Weight Loss

When my husband, kids and I moved to Kentucky in June of 2000, I stood very calmly in the Department of Motor Vehicles and told a spectacular lie. Now, I normally consider myself to be an honest person. But, one major, ironclad, cast in stone, no doubt about it, "Rule of Life" is that no one tells the truth when someone asks about weight.

We all know that we're going to lie. And the heavier you are, the bigger the lie. How many pounds can you deny without the person behind the counter breaking into hysterical laughter? I opted for a verbal weight loss of 72 pounds. The woman behind the counter put 175 pounds on my license without batting an eyelash. Bless her kind soul.

What should my license have read? Birth date: 10/18/52. Height: 5'2".
Weight: 247 pounds. What did these vital statistics reveal?

- 47 years old.
- Short.
- Fat.

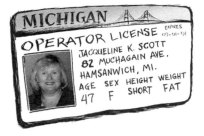

I didn't mind being 47. I was used to being short. I hated being fat. And
I was fat enough to meet the medical definition of morbid obesity — 100
pounds over "normal" weight.

When I was lying about my weight at the Department of Motor Vehicles,
I easily could have been included in the overweight women study. I weighed
247 pounds, and my dream weight coincided with theirs — 135 pounds.
That weight represented a 45 percent reduction in body weight, and, coin-
cidentally, corresponded with the medical definition of normal weight for
my height. I needed to lose a mere 112 pounds in order to satisfy the dream
of being thin.

The justification for my lie was easy; I was starting a new diet, so it was
just a matter of time before the weight on my license was correct. Perfectly
reasonable logic. Based on the logic of that statement, I started thinking
about the last time the weight on my driver's license was accurate.

When I was a senior in college, I gained 20 pounds my final semester. I
had stupidly signed up to take organic chemistry pass-fail. I had more cred-
it hours than I needed to graduate, but I needed a three-hour science elec-
tive. My husband, Brett, was a chemical engineering major, so I thought it
would be nice if I learned a little organic chemistry. This was not a wise decision on my part and a little was exactly how much I learned. By the time I
survived the course, and somehow made a C, I weighed 147 pounds. It was
the most I had ever weighed. I would never have believed that one day I'd
weigh 100 pounds more.

In the summer of 1974, I joined Weight Watchers® for the first time and I lost 35 pounds. Therefore, sometime in the fall of 1974, I would have weighed what my driver's license said I did. So, it had been 27 years since my license weight had been correct.

The worst part of this story is that even when I weighed 112 pounds, I wasn't happy with my body. I still looked bad in shorts because my thighs were not perfectly proportioned with the rest of my body. My fingernails hadn't miraculously become long and strong. No photographer appeared, begging me to participate in a photo shoot featuring Women of the Big Ten. I was thinner than I'd been since fifth grade, and I still wasn't happy with my body.

The Dream of Physical Perfection

The dream represents more than just being thin; the dream represents physical perfection. A great body is just the beginning. Women also want flawless makeup, an excellent manicure and thick, shiny, manageable hair. Men want muscular chests, flat stomachs, and enough hair so their scalp doesn't show through. We all want to be attractive, and we're willing to consider injections, liposuction, and surgery in our search for external beauty.

Why do we do this to ourselves? Why do we insist on comparing ourselves to the limited and unrealistic perspective presented by Hollywood and Madison Avenue? Based on the height, size and weight of the average woman, there has never been a greater difference between the women chosen to represent us and ourselves. And even though we know it, we still blame ourselves rather than the people responsible for creating this disparity.

Societal influences contribute greatly to our unrealistic expectations of appropriate weights and body shapes. Television and print ads surround us with images of disgustingly young, amazingly tall, impossibly thin women. Oh yeah, and it's not enough that they're young and tall and thin, they're also gorgeous and have high, firm, full breasts. Where do they find these women? Are they cloning them in the basements of New York modeling agencies? Are they grown on specially grafted trees in a top-secret research facility high in the Beverly Hills?

Trust me, these women are NOT average. Remember, the average woman is 5'4" tall, weighs 148 pounds and wears a size 14. How does she compare to the average model? The average high-fashion model is 5'10", 117 pounds and wears a size 4 or 6. The only thing that the average woman has in common with the average model is that neither is happy with her weight. They're both on a diet.

When we lose weight, we're devastated to discover that losing weight simply produces a smaller version of our less-than-perfect bodies. We can wear a smaller size. We look better in clothing. But, we still look crummy in a bathing suit.

Who should we blame? Fairy tales or television or movies? Have we spent so much time looking at unrealistically beautiful people that we can no longer recognize normal? Quit watching TV. Go to the mall, to the grocery store, to the discount store. Look around. This is what normal looks like. And normal is okay.

Are we doomed to be shallow and unhappy? If we find a genie's bottle washed up on the beach, will we ask for thin thighs or world peace? If we catch a leprechaun perched on a rainbow, do six-pack abs seem more important than a cure for AIDS?

Focus On the Possible

If you want to lose weight and keep it off, you have to start making changes in your head. When you decide to diet, do so with realistic expectations. Losing weight changes a number on the scales. It may make you happier and healthier; it won't make you perfect.

If you're a 100 pounds overweight, it's easy to decide that you need to lose weight. But the question is not necessarily easy to answer if you're 10, 20 or even 40 pounds heavier than the recommended weight for your height.

If you're 50, and you're still trying to weigh what you did when you were twenty, you're expecting a lot. If you're a reasonable weight, if your blood pressure is normal, if you're not diabetic, and your cholesterol and triglycerides are in the normal range, maybe you should quit worrying about the scales and start walking for a half hour every day.

Before you decide to go on a diet, make sure that your present weight isn't acceptable for your current age and stage of life. If you do decide to go on a diet, focus on becoming a healthy weight and getting some exercise. Focus on what's possible.

Accept the fact that your thighs are not going to be thin. Consider the possibility that it doesn't matter. It's not only mentally unhealthy to set completely unrealistic goals, it also makes losing weight and keeping it off much more difficult.

chapter 2

Searching for the Perfect Diet

Since you purchased this book, there's a good chance you're overweight or obese. You're not alone. The government keeps lots of statistics on health and nutrition and the most recently published results have focused tremendous attention on the nation's epidemic of obesity. According to statistics from the 1994 and 1999 National Health and Nutrition Examination Surveys (NHANES), the number of overweight people in the present population increased six percent, from 55 percent to 61 percent, in only five years.

In June 2000, Diane, my daughter, and I fit nicely into the national statistics, but we didn't fit nicely into anything else. Diane needed to lose more than 200 pounds. I needed to lose at least 100 pounds.

If I lost 100 pounds, I could move out of the Land of the Morbidly Obese into the slim trim neighborhood of the Merely Overweight. The loss of 100 pounds would put me at a weight of 147 pounds.

This was a weight that had been one of my weight plateaus (before I moved on to weight mountains). It was what I weighed at age twenty-two, when I joined Weight Watchers® the first time. It was what I weighed each of the two times I became pregnant. It was the lowest weight I achieved after each pregnancy.

It was also a weight I hadn't seen in about fifteen years, but losing 100 pounds sounded nice. No, it sounded great. But, honestly, when we started this, I thought if I ever got below 200 pounds I'd be ecstatic. I made a commitment to my husband, my daughter and myself to try one more time to lose weight. But that was it. One more time was all I had left in me.

Diet Failures

I'd spent the last twenty years dieting and I'd spent those twenty years getting fatter and fatter. My previous diet efforts had obviously not provided a long-term answer to my weight problems.

By analyzing and categorizing our previous diet failures, we identified certain patterns, which in turn, helped us avoid the same mistakes this time around.

When did our diets fail?

Some diets failed us at the beginning. Those were the diets that either allowed so little food or placed such restrictions on the food permitted, that we never stayed on the diet long enough to lose any significant amount of weight.

Some diets failed us at the end. We lost weight, but we gained it back. Sometimes we gained it back slowly. Sometimes we gained it back quickly. But we always gained it back.

Why did our diets fail?

The diets that failed us in the beginning failed due to our mind's response to our dieting choices. We were bombarded by promises of fast and easy weight loss, so we started each new diet with the same unrealistic expectations. At the beginning of the diet, when weight loss was rapid (due primarily to the loss of water), we did well. As soon as weight loss slowed, we became discouraged and quit. We hadn't mentally prepared ourselves to make any permanent and sustainable changes in our diet.

The diets that failed us at the end failed due to our body's response to dieting. Diets restrict calories in order to maximize the rate of weight loss, but extremely restrictive diets are interpreted by the body as evidence of famine. Since the body does not distinguish between self-induced famine and the real thing, it responds to low calorie diets by decreasing the body's energy requirements, depleting stored protein and reducing muscle mass.

Since fat is the least metabolically active tissue, it is the least affected by the decreased energy provided by a low calorie diet. It becomes increasingly difficult to lose weight, despite the low calorie intake. People are literally starving themselves with no results to show for it. A recent study indicated that a 200-pound woman limited to an 800 calorie a day diet might experience a 15 percent decline in metabolic rate after only three weeks.

Once dieting stops and normal eating resumes, the weight gain is accelerated due to the decrease in metabolism. Even worse, during the dieting phase, the body has lost muscle mass; during weight gaining, the body regains fat. When weight is regained, the dieter has a higher percentage of body fat. Since fat metabolizes fewer calories than muscle, the same weight is actually sustained by fewer calories.

Once we determined that our previous diets had failed due to our body's normal psychological and physical reaction to dieting, we began to itemize the requirements of the perfect diet. The diet that wouldn't fail us at the beginning. The diet that wouldn't fail us at the end. The diet we could stay on a really long time. The diet that would keep the weight off.

The Perfect Diet

Once we knew exactly what we were looking for, we began searching diligently for that perfect diet. I started at the library and at the new and used bookstores. There's a never-ending supply of diet books, so Brett, my husband, and I read new ones and old ones, million copy sellers and one print wonders. I highlighted and took notes, and I asked Brett question after question.

What did we discover? In the lucrative world of diet books, the same information and misinformation keeps getting recycled, repackaged, relabeled and resold. There are lots of diets out there, but many of the supposedly new ideas are just minor variations on old themes. And some of these old ideas were conceived when our knowledge and understanding of physiology and nutrition were tremendously limited.

Non-traditional diet books present ideas that differ from the traditional medical community's opinions on health and nutrition, and explain the conflict by indicating that they are privy to information the rest of the medical community is lacking. These books frequently contain elaborate explanations for their personal diet theory, but underneath a lot of pseudo-scientific explanations designed to impress and intimidate readers, the basic rules of thermodynamics have not changed. Diets work when your caloric intake is less than your caloric expenditure. This basic fact is frequently disguised by elaborate rules for what to eat, when to eat it and what to eat it with. But if you cut through the camouflage, you end up with a reduced calorie diet, just in disguise. And frequently it's a diet that is not nutritionally balanced due to the restrictions placed on the consumption of certain food groups.

Traditional diets place no restrictions on types of foods, they simply reduce daily caloric intake in order to achieve weight loss. Since many nutrition experts believe it is very difficult to consume adequate nutrients at these caloric levels, these diets are often referred to as semi-starvation diets. Most of us have had personal experience with the accuracy of this description. It is very difficult to eat the calorie allotment of the typical reduced-calorie diet without feeling physically hungry, bodily fatigued and mentally deprived.

The more I read, the more convinced I became that winning the losing game would require a different approach. Why was I fat despite years of dieting? I didn't need to learn to diet. I needed to learn to eat.

Most diets focus on losing weight, but overweight is not the problem. It's the symptom of the problem. What's the problem? The problem is poor eating habits.

If someone loses weight by going on a diet, but doesn't make permanent changes in their eating habits, they're wasting their time. As soon as they quit dieting and return to their old eating habits, they regain the weight. The goal of a diet should be learning how to eat properly.

Once I had identified my goal, I defined it.

What is proper eating?
Proper eating is consuming a nutritious, well-balanced variety of foods in proper portions that maintain a healthy weight.

After I identified and defined my goal, I needed to put it into action. Where does one go to learn to eat properly? Based on the present national statistics, The School of Proper Eating appears to be closed. Or is it?

Another look at those statistics shows that in addition to the 61 percent of the population that is overweight or obese, three percent are classified as underweight. Do a little math and you discover that 36 percent of the population is presently maintaining a weight classified as normal.

Inspiration struck. In order to be a normal weight, I needed to learn to eat like someone who already was a normal weight. In my case, I needed to know what the 5'2" female who maintained a weight of 135 pounds was eating. I needed to learn to eat like her.

The goal of *Eucalorics* is to teach you to eat like the normal weight person you wish to become.

chapter 3

Eucalories

Why eucaloric? The prefix *eu* means normal, so an eucaloric diet is a normal calorie diet. It is a diet designed to achieve and maintain a normal weight by consistently consuming the number of calories that support a normal weight.

What is a normal weight? How is it defined?

What we refer to as a normal weight is actually a range of weights that corresponds to BMI's (body mass indices) between 18.5 and 24.9. The correlation between BMI's and weight categories is summarized in Table 3.1.

< 18.5	Underweight
18.5 - 24.9	Normal Weight
25.0 - 29.9	Overweight
30.0 - 34.9	Obese I (Mild)
35.0 - 39.9	Obese II (Moderate)
40.0 - 44.9	Obese III (Extreme)
> 45.0	Obese IV (Morbid)

Table 3.1 Weight Categories

Table 3.2 contains a chart based on BMI calculations. Body mass indices are determined using the following mathematical formula:

$$BMI = (\text{Weight in pounds}/(\text{Height in inches})^2) \times 704.5$$

Table 3.2 presents the results of that formula as a graph. The range of normal weights for my height, 5'2" or 62", is highlighted.

HEIGHT	NORMAL	OVERWEIGHT	OBESE I	OBESE II	OBESE III	OBESE IV
58	88-118	119-142	143-166	167-190	191-214	over 214
59	91-123	124-147	148-172	173-196	197-222	over 222
60	95-127	128-152	153-178	179-203	204-229	over 229
61	98-131	132-157	158-184	185-210	211-237	over 237
62	101-135	136-163	164-190	191-217	218-245	over 245
63	104-140	141-168	169-196	197-224	225-253	over 253
64	108-144	145-173	174-202	203-231	232-261	over 261
65	111-149	150-181	180-219	210-238	239-269	over 269
66	114-154	155-184	185-215	216-246	247-278	over 278
67	118-158	159-190	191-222	223-253	254-286	over 286
68	121-163	164-196	197-229	230-261	262-295	over 295
69	125-168	169-202	203-236	237-269	270-303	over 303
70	129-173	174-208	209-242	243-277	278-312	over 312
71	132-178	179-214	215-249	250-285	286-321	over 321
72	136-183	184-220	221-257	258-293	294-330	over 330
73	140-188	189-226	227-264	265-301	302-340	over 340
74	144-193	194-232	233-271	272-309	310-349	over 349
75	148-199	200-239	240-278	279-318	319-358	over 358
76	152-204	205-246	246-286	287-326	327-368	over 368

Table 3.2 Body Mass Index Weight Ranges

Normal weight for my height ranges from 101-135 pounds. My dream weight, 135 pounds, is the highest weight that still places me in the normal weight category.

How many calories does it take to sustain my dream weight?

According to research physiologists, an inactive female can maintain weight by consuming 12 calories per pound of body weight. That number is based on 10 calories per pound for basic metabolic processes such as breathing and cell maintenance, and two calories per pound for walking to the refrigerator, pushing the buttons on the remote, and shopping for junk food. An inactive male gets 14 calories per pound to maintain weight. These extra calories are due primarily to the increased muscle mass in males.

It is worth noting that the 12 calorie/pound and 14 calorie/pound numbers calculations are most accurate for normal weights. Since fat is relatively metabolically inactive, it takes fewer calories to sustain fat than to sustain lean muscle mass. The higher the percentage of fat represented by our body composition, the less accurate the numbers become. Based on my own personal weight loss history, the 12 calorie/pound number is a reasonable estimate, and we use that estimate in all our calculations.

If I want to weigh 135 pounds, I calculate my daily caloric intake as follows:

135 pounds x 12 calorie/pound = 1,620 calories

In order to maintain a weight of 135 pounds, I can eat 1,620 calories each day. More specifically, in order to maintain a weight of 135 pounds, I *have* to average 1,620 calories each day.

If I routinely eat fewer calories, I'll lose weight. If I routinely eat more calories, I'll gain weight.

In order to weigh 135 pounds, I have to be mentally and physically happy eating the number of calories that sustains that weight. Every day. Day after day. Forever.

In order to weigh 135 pounds, I started eating as if I already did. I started eating 1,600 calories a day.

How do you learn to follow a Eucaloric Diet?
To get started, you pick a weight. Calculate how many calories it takes to sustain that weight. Start eating that number of calories. Don't stop.

Wait a minute. You expect me to believe you and Diane lost three hundred pounds eating 1,600 calorie a day? That's not possible.

If you're reading this book and you're female, there's a reasonably good chance that your dream weight is the same as my dream weight, 135 pounds. It's difficult to believe that it's possible to lose weight eating 1,600 calories a day, because you've never been able to lose weight eating 1,000-1,200 calories a day. How can you possibly lose weight eating so many calories?

You have to be willing to make one extremely significant change in the way you approach weight loss.

When people find out I've lost a hundred pounds, the first question they invariably ask is, "How long did it take you?"

I've got a standard answer. I always tell people, "You're asking the wrong question."

OK. What is the right question?

How long have you kept the weight off?

What possible difference does it make how long it took me to lose weight, if in the process of losing it I've learned to keep it off?

I was an experienced participant in the weight loss game. I tried every new diet. I bought books and magazines. I knew about carbohydrate addictions and sugar allergies. I watched infomercials. I read about zones and counting points, and, despite all my efforts, I'd spent the last twenty years getting fatter and fatter.

What does *Eucalorics* require for success? You have to quit worshipping at the altar of quick weight loss. Advertising quick weight loss may sell diet books and a truly astonishing number of "miracle" diet pills, but it's not doing a thing for teaching us, the overweight population, how to lose weight and keep it off.

Eucalorics isn't about losing weight quickly. It's about losing weight forever. It's about accepting responsibility for your present weight problems and learning to make permanent changes in your life that will allow you to achieve and maintain a normal weight

Accepting Responsibility

No one wants to be overweight, but as we struggle and fail at losing weight, it's easy to be seduced by any explanation that allows us to blame our obesity on factors which are not in our control. Bestselling diet books are filled with elaborate theories for why we're overweight. They tell us we eat the wrong types of food, we eat the wrong combinations of food, we eat incorrectly for our blood type, we metabolize insulin improperly, or we eat at the wrong time of year.

We need to realize that it has not helped us to blame our weight on someone or something other than ourselves. Before we can solve our weight problems, we have to identify the problem and we have to start by admitting some unpleasant truths. Why is everyone fat? Because we eat too much and exercise too little.

Yuck. We hate that answer.

You want a different answer? OK.

Everyone is fat because their caloric intake is more than their caloric expenditure.

That's not fair. It's the same answer, just dressed up a little to be polite.

Sorry. If you want a different answer, buy a different book. There are lots to choose from. When we typed diet into the search engine at *Amazon.com*, there were 30,000 books in the database. These books are filled with scientifically complicated, but polite explanations for overweight. In these books, dieting theories are difficult, but once you understand *their* particular theory, dieting is supposed to be easy.

In real life, when you put the book on the coffee table and walk into the kitchen, the reverse is true. Theoretical dieting may be easy, but actual dieting is hard. It's time to stop dieting and start learning to eat. It's time to learn new habits.

The first critical step in learning new habits is admitting the truth about our old habits. Why were we fat? We didn't have metabolic disorders, and we weren't allergic to carbohydrates. Our thyroids were functioning and our pancreases were doing a fine job producing insulin. Why were we fat? We were victims of overactive fork disease, and our tennis shoes never played tennis. We ate too much and exercised too little.

Traditional diets promote weight loss based on the body's energy equation. What does this equation look like?

Caloric intake = base metabolism + physical activity = Caloric expenditure

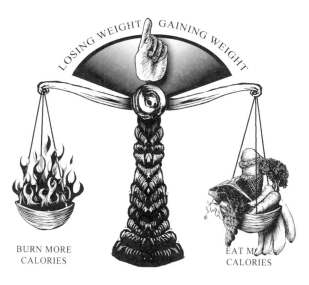

BURN MORE
CALORIES

EAT MORE
CALORIES

When our bodies are in a state of caloric equilibrium, our caloric intake equals our caloric expenditure, and we maintain weight.

If our caloric intake is less than our caloric expenditure, we lose weight. We're eating an insufficient number of calories.

If our caloric intake is greater than our caloric expenditure, we gain weight. We're eating an excessive number of calories.

Each pound of stored fat represents 3,500 calories of potential energy. In order to lose a pound of fat, we have to be calorically "out-of-balance" by a deficit of 3,500 calories. Since caloric expenditure is a combination of basic metabolic processes and exercise, we can lose weight either by reducing caloric intake or by increasing our exercise level or both.

Traditional diets generally prescribe daily caloric intakes of 1,000-1,200 calories per day. And people *do* lose weight on low-calorie diets. The problem is that when people stop dieting, they gain all the weight back.

The failure of traditional diets to maintain weight loss led to the proliferation of non-traditional diets described in a never-ending variety of *diet de jour* weight loss books. Just as people lost weight on traditional low-calorie diets, people lose weight on these diets also. The problem with all diets is when people stop dieting, they gain all the weight back.

If we do not make permanent sustainable changes in our eating habits while losing weight, we have very little chance of maintaining that weight loss.

The best way to create new habits is to start to do the same thing over and over. Every day. Day after day. Forever.

If you want to be a specific weight, calculate how many calories it takes to maintain that weight. Start to eat to maintain that weight. Every day. Day after day. Forever.

Stop worrying about losing weight quickly. Start concentrating on losing weight permanently by learning new eating habits.

People with weight problems know how to diet. We know how to overeat. We know how to starve. We know how to binge. We don't know how to eat properly. Instead of spending our lives on an endless cycle of dieting and binging, losing and gaining, we need to achieve and maintain a healthy weight by learning to eat properly.

How did I lose so much weight? I started eating 1,600 calories a day. Day after day. I lost weight. I continued to lose weight, but I lost weight more and more slowly. Eventually my weight loss stopped. I continued to eat 1.600 calories a day. Nothing else changed.

Eucalorics is based on the premise that weight loss should occur as a result of eating properly, as a result of eating the number of calories that will support a normal weight. *Eucalorics* isn't a traditional diet that signifigantly restricts calories in order to lose weight. *Eucalorics* isn't a non-traditional diet that relies on complicated rules about what to eat or when to eat. *Eucalorics* is a weight maintenance program. Maintenance starts the first day. Weight loss happens while you're practicing maintenance.

When you reach your goal weight, weight loss stops. You keep practicing maintenance. One day you look around and you're not practicing maintenance any more, you're just maintaining.

chapter 4

A Different Approach

The hardest part about *Eucalorics* isn't the diet. It's getting people to believe the diet works. It sounds too easy to be a real diet.

We probably couldn't get anyone to listen to our uncomplicated theories if it wasn't for the amazing amount of weight that we've lost. When you lose 100 pounds and keep it off or 200 pounds and keep it off, it becomes rather difficult for anyone to say your theories can't possibly work.

People ask us about weight loss all the time. Lose three hundred pounds and trust me, people become very interested. We give them the same embarrassingly easy explanation we gave you.

Pick a weight. Multiple that weight by 12 (or 14). Start eating that number of calories. Don't stop.

What makes this diet easier to follow? If you choose a sensible goal weight, you'll get to eat more food.

When we start a typical reduced-calorie diet, we switch from normal eating mode to diet eating mode. The rules of diet eating are easy. If you like it, you can't have it. If it tastes good, you can't have it. If it's on a menu, you can't have it. What do you get to eat when you're on a diet? Grilled chicken. Lettuce. Meals in cans. Frozen dinners.

Why is it so hard to stay on most diets? *YOU'RE ALWAYS HUNGRY.* If you try to lose weight on a traditional diet, you're going to be hungry. Diets routinely have people consuming 1,000 to 1,200 calories per day, but it's impossible to be happy eating this number of calories. Why? There's actually a pretty simple explanation. Do a little math and the reason becomes obvious; you're not eating enough food.

What weight does 1,000 calories a day support?

Female:

$$\frac{1,000 \text{ calories}}{12 \text{ calories/pound}} = 83 \text{ pounds}$$

Male:

$$\frac{1,000 \text{ calories}}{14 \text{ calories/pound}} = 71 \text{ pounds}$$

No wonder you're hungry. If you're female, you're only eating enough calories to support an 83-pound woman; if you're male, you're only eating enough calories to support a 71-pound man.

If you're on some type of muscle-sparing protein supplement diet that provides as little as 600 calories a day, the numbers are even worse.

What weight does 600 calories a day support?

Female:

$$\frac{600 \text{ calories}}{12 \text{ calories/pound}} = 50 \text{ pounds}$$

Male:

$$\frac{600 \text{ calories}}{14 \text{ calories/pound}} = 43 \text{ pounds}$$

With this amount of calories, you're only eating enough food to support a 50-pound woman or a 43-pound man. It's no wonder your body thinks the famine has arrived. It has. Your metabolic rate is decreasing and your body is trying desperately to reduce your energy requirements.

I don't want to weigh 83 pounds. So, why do I try to lose weight by eating to support a weight of 83 pounds? We don't need to learn to diet. We need to learn to eat properly. Eating 1,000 calories a day isn't eating properly. Eating properly is eating a well-balanced, nutritional variety of foods that will support a healthy weight.

It is possible to sabotage *Eucalorics* by picking a goal weight that is extremely difficult to attain. When you decide to pick a goal weight, give yourself a fighting chance. You're allowed to pick a dream weight, but you need to stay away from fantasy weights.

What's the difference?

A dream weight is possible. It may be a long way away, it may be ambitious, but it's possible. *A fantasy weight requires a plane crash on a remote desert island.*

There are numerous other charts, graphs and calculations that are used to establish desirable weights other than BMI. For some reason, it's difficult for us to resist picking the system that places us at the lowest possible weight. My fantasy weight system allows 100 pounds for the first five feet of height and five pounds for each additional inch of height. According to that calculation, I should weigh 110 pounds.

There's obviously been at least one day in my life when I weighed 110 pounds, but I have no idea which day it was. Maybe it was only part of a day. Maybe I was an infant. Still, I love the idea of weighing 110 pounds. There's just one question. Which limb am I willing to sacrifice to do so?

Still not convinced? Let's use that BMI calculation and do a little math.

$$BMI = (Weight\ in\ pounds/(Height\ in\ inches)^2) \times 704.5$$

Let's use this formula and take a look at the people in New York City and Hollywood that we keep comparing ourselves to.

For example, the high-fashion model. She's unbelievably tall: 5'10". She's incredibly thin: 117 pounds. What's her BMI?

$$BMI = (Weight\ in\ pounds/(Height\ in\ inches)^2) \times 704.5$$

$$BMI = (117\ /(70)^2) \times 704.5$$
$$= (117\ /4900) \times 704.5$$
$$= (0.024) \times 704.5$$
$$= 16.9$$

Her BMI is significantly less than 18.5; at 117 pounds, she's clearly underweight.

Let's put this in perspective. What would I have to weigh to have a BMI of 16.9? What would my BMI have to be in order for me to look like this model? We start with the BMI formula.

$$\text{BMI} = (\text{Weight in pounds}/(\text{Height in inches})^2) \times 704.5$$

We solve for weight in pounds.

$$
\begin{aligned}
\textbf{Weight in pounds} &= (\text{BMI}/704.5)(\text{height in inches})^2 \\
&= (16.9/704.5)(62)^2 \\
&= (.024)(3844) \\
&= \textbf{92 pounds}
\end{aligned}
$$

I'd have to weigh 92 pounds to have a BMI of 16.9. I think I last weighed 92 pounds in the third grade. What would I get to eat in order to maintain that weight?

$$\textbf{92 pounds} \times \textbf{12 calories/pound/day} = \textbf{1,104 calories/day}$$

Suppose I somehow arrive at a weight of 92 pounds. (I've been locked in a closet for eight months and fed two crackers and bottled water once a day by a crazed fashion magazine cameraman.) When I escape from the closet, I get to gorge myself on 1,100 calories a day for the rest of time in order to maintain my new weight. Hmmm. Ninety-two pounds is not looking good.

Okay, I'm actually eight inches too short to be a high-fashion model but what if I'm willing to settle for becoming a star of the stage and/or screen? (We'll be polite and ignore my age.) Most Hollywood stars have heights and weights that classify them as underweight, a BMI below 18.5. I'm willing to be a rather plump star, so I'm going to aim for a BMI of exactly 18.5.

$$
\begin{aligned}
\textbf{Weight in pounds} &= (\text{BMI}/704.5)(\text{height in inches})^2 \\
&= (18.5/704.5)(62)^2 \\
&= (.026)(3844) \\
&= \textbf{100 pounds}
\end{aligned}
$$

What do I get to eat, if I weigh 100 pounds?

100 pounds x 12 calories/pound = 1,200 calories/day

Wait. That number sounds familiar. Oh, yeah. I've tried eating 1,200 calories a day; it is the high end of the semi-starvation diet. I was miserable eating 1,200 calories a day.

Remember my fantasy weight? 110 pounds, right? We already established that I'm never going to weigh 110 pounds. It simply isn't going to happen. If I'm never going to weigh 110 pounds, does it make sense for me to try to diet by eating the number of calories that sustains a weight even lower than my fantasy weight? A weight that I will never reach or maintain?

But, that's exactly how most diets work. Most diets reduce daily caloric intake to significantly less than it takes to maintain our goal weights in order to promote quick weight loss. We're hungry and we're miserable, because we're trying to exist on the calories that will maintain unreasonable weights.

We either don't stay on the diets long enough to lose much weight or if we do lose weight, we gain the weight back. We haven't made any long-term changes to our eating habits, so we don't know how to maintain our weight loss once we get there. The diets either fail us at the beginning or fail us at the end.

I decided that the weight of a model or Hollywood starlet shouldn't be my goal. Maybe it shouldn't be your goal. Remember, these people are not the norm. Do yourself a favor and pick a reasonable goal. Don't doom yourself to failure by selecting a BMI goal for which less than three percent of the population qualifies. Pick a reasonable goal. It can always be changed.

If you're obese, start with the goal of becoming overweight. If you're overweight or lose enough weight to become overweight, you can decide to aim for a normal weight. Remember, *you have to be mentally and physically happy eating the number of calories that will support the weight you have chosen.*

Take a look at the goal weight you picked. Did you pick that weight by asking, what do I want to weigh? Take a look at the number of calories that will maintain that weight and ask a different question. Is this a weight you can live with once you get there? A weight you can live with involves being willing and happy to eat the number of calories it takes to sustain that weight every day.

Sound too simplistic? It is somewhat simplistic. Excess caloric intake can be balanced with physical activity. (Physical activity would be exercise for those of us who aren't familiar with that particular phrase.) The 12-calorie per pound number is based on a relatively inactive lifestyle. Start exercising and you get to eat more food. For the moment, we'll assume you are presently inactive and the 12-calorie per pound or 14-calorie per pound number is a good starting point. Why do we make that assumption? Since only 15 percent of adults presently meet the government recommendations of regular moderate physical activity for at least 30 minutes per day, it seems to be a reasonable assumption to make.

My goal was the highest weight that would still place me in the normal weight category. This weight allows me to eat 1,620 calories a day. It's a dream weight, not a fantasy weight.

Ready to pick a weight? Fill in the chart below and then calculate your daily caloric allotment. If you're female, multiply that weight by 12. If you're male, multiply that weight by 14.

Goal Weight in pounds = _____ .

Female

_____ x 12 calories/pound/day = _____ calories/day
Weight in pounds

Male

_____ x 14 calories/pound/day = _____ calories/day
Weight in pounds

You've picked a goal weight and determined your daily caloric allotment. Now it's time to start paying attention to what you eat. It's time to start developing new eating habits and learning to achieve and maintain your goal weight. It's time to start learning to eat properly.

chapter 5

New Habits

The goal of *Eucalorics* is not simply weight loss, it's permanent weight loss. Permanent weight loss can only be achieved by making permanent changes in our daily fare, our diet. In order to make permanent changes in our daily fare we need to learn new habits.

The solution to bad eating habits is different than the solution to most other bad habits. The message for most bad habits is simple. Stop. If you smoke, stop smoking. If you bite your fingernails, stop biting them. If you drink to excess, stop drinking. If you have a drug problem, stop taking drugs. The cure for most bad habits is to stop the problem behavior completely.

Diets are the equivalent to the stop solution to a bad habit. Stop eating carbohydrates. Stop eating protein. Stop eating fat. Stop eating. But the stop solution doesn't work for food, because not eating is not compatible with continued life and health. Bad eating habits require change. These poor food relationships need to be replaced with good eating habits and the key to developing new habits is repetition.

As long as my caloric consumption averages 1,600 calories a day, I won't gain weight. I could eat 800 calories one day and 2,400 calories the next day. I would maintain my weight, but I would not be developing good eating habits. The best way to learn new eating habits is to eat consistently. Eat the same number of calories every day. The more consistently you eat, the more habitual this new pattern of eating will become. When we eat properly and consistently, our bodies become used to eating the correct number of calories in the proper portions.

I've changed not only what I eat, but also how I eat. I try very hard to eat consistently, because eating consistently makes it easier to eat properly.

Before we designed *Eucalorics*, we were following a traditional reduced-calorie diet and I was eating 1,200 calories a day. I was losing weight, but I was miserable. I knew I'd never be able to continue this type of diet long-term. When I started eating 1,600 calories a day, it became much easier to stay on a diet. Increasing my daily calories from 1,200 calories to 1,600 calories represented a 33 percent increase in caloric intake.

Keep in mind the *reason that diets fail in the beginning* — because they allow so little food or place such restrictions on the types of food, that we never stay on the diet long enough to lose any weight. This is not brain surgery. It's easier to stay on a diet when you get more food.

What about losing weight?

One of the most difficult things for us to convince people is they can lose weight while eating well. Everyone believes that losing weight, i.e. dieting, means eating horrible food and being hungry all the time.

If you are overweight and begin to eat properly, you will begin to lose weight. The heavier you are, the quicker you will lose weight. If you exercise, you will lose weight even faster. In June 2000, I weighed 247 pounds. How many calories did it take to maintain that weight?

247 pounds x 12 calories/pound/day = 2,964 calories/day

My instinctive reaction to that number was a quick side trip into the Land of Denial. There was no way I was consuming almost 3,000 calories per day. Or was I? My usual fast food feast consisted of a batter-dipped and fried chicken breast with dressing on a bun. It was accompanied by french fries, a medium chocolate dairy dessert, and, of course, a diet drink.

How many calories was I eating? Would you believe 1,310 calories and 45 grams of fat? If I'm trying to weigh 135 pounds, I just ate 78 percent of my daily calories for lunch.

CHICKEN SANDWICH	430 calories	15 fat grams
LARGE FRIES	440 calories	19 fat grams
DAIRY DESSERT	440 calories	11 fat grams
GRAND TOTAL:	1310 calories	45 fat grams

Table 5.1

What about my personal favorite food, ice cream? It's packed in pint-sized cartons whose small print mentions something about four servings. Yeah, right. My all-time favorite flavor, chocolate chip cookie dough has 1,080 calories and 68 grams of fat in each carton and I never picked up a pint without eating the entire carton. If I was having a bad day, that pint of ice cream was frequently consumed with a package of cookies.

I decided to consider the possibility that I was averaging almost 3,000 calories per day. Since I was eating that many calories each day, I didn't have to reduce my calories to starvation level in order to lose weight.

When I was eating 1,200 calories a day, I was losing weight. When I started eating 1,620 calories a day, I still lost weight. Would I have lost weight more quickly on 1,200 calories a day? It depends. When I started eating 1,620 calories, I was getting more food, so I stayed on the diet.

Weight loss eating 1,200 calories.
(2,964 – 1,200) calories/day = 1,764 calories/day
3,500 calories/pound /1,764 calories/day= 1.98 days/pound
7 days/week/1.98 days/pound = 3.5 pounds/week

Weight loss eating 1,620 calories.
(2,964 – 1,620) calories/day = 1,344 calories/day
3,500 calories/pound /1,344 calories/day= 2.6 days/pound
7 days/week/2.6 days/pound = 2.7 pounds/week

Not too surprisingly, weight loss is more rapid on a semi-starvation diet, but the difference is less than a pound a week. Am I willing to exchange a pound a week in weight loss for 33 percent more food? You bet I am. Especially since I rarely stayed on a low-calorie diet long enough to lose any meaningful amount of weight. In addition, the feelings of deprivation associated with a semi-starvation diet usually led to binging behavior and weight gain.

If you begin to consistently eat the calories that will support your goal weight, you will discover how much easier it is to eat sensibly when you aren't hungry all the time. It's easier, but it is still difficult to eat properly in today's world. In order to eat properly, you need to become an educated consumer. The more knowledge you possess, the better the food choices you can make. You need to know as much as possible about food processing and preparation. You need to understand the psychology that influences your choices. You need to be prepared.

You're about to start making permanent changes in the way you eat. Permanent changes in the way you view food. It is possible. It is not always easy, but, it's worth the effort.

I had spent most of my adult life unhappy about my weight and miserable around food. I didn't control my eating; my eating controlled me. Every Monday morning I started another diet. And every time I started and failed, I was miserable. Food was the one aspect of my life over which I seemed to have no control and I hated it.

Eucalorics gave me the control that I needed in order to make permanent changes in my life. Learning to eat properly gave me the ability to deal with my own personal diet demons, the foods that I ate to excess, the foods I binged on. The foods that I associated with another diet failure.

The frustrations associated with yo-yo dieting have warped our attitudes toward food. Food is no longer viewed as the provider of either simple nourishment or gastronomic pleasure, but as an all-powerful entity with a combination of abstract and human characteristics. It is viewed as good or bad. It is labeled legal or illegal.

Diane and I learned to accept that food is simply food. That no one comes to arrest us if we eat a cookie. An open bag of chocolate is not a sign of deep moral decay. Bad food is the food in the back of the refrigerator with mold growing on it, or chicken salad with mayonnaise sitting overnight on the counter.

Eating properly does not focus on fat-free food or carbohydrate-free food; eating properly focuses on guilt-free food. There are no bad foods. There are no illegal foods. Some foods are low fat and low calorie. Some foods are high fat and high calorie. It's all just food. This thought is accompanied by the following valuable information: It is highly unlikely that any food available today will not be available tomorrow. It is not necessary or recommended to try to eat every piece of candy or all of the cookies today. They'll make more.

When any food is labeled bad, it's human nature to instantly want it. When we begin eating these bad foods, we don't just eat, we binge. We eat until the bag or box is empty. As long as there is bad food around, we are subject to continued temptation. In order for us to be restored to good behavior, the bad food must all be consumed. The knowledge that all food is permitted, appears to be a critical element in eliminating the feelings of guilt that frequently initiate and accompany binging.

I have lost a tremendous amount of weight, but the weight loss is not the best thing that happened. Somewhere along the way, I learned to eat two cookies from a package that contained twenty. I learned to eat two cookies today, and two cookies tomorrow, and two cookies the next day. When you eat the box two cookies at a time, you get to enjoy eating cookies without feeling guilty about eating them. This is a big deal. When was the last time you ate cookies without feeling guilty? Since I went on my first diet when I was eleven, I had probably eaten my last guilt-free cookie when I was ten.

The ability to accept food as just food is important in developing a healthy relationship with it. It is more important to have learned to eat two cookies, than to have lost weight, because learning to eat two cookies is what makes maintaining my weight loss possible. I've lost weight before. I never learned to eat two cookies before.

If you don't learn to eat at fast food and fancy restaurants, and to eat candy, cookies and chips, you may lose weight, but you have little chance of keeping the weight off.

You need to learn to live with food, not without it, in order to lose weight permanently!

I am sincerely and intensely devoted to chocolate chip cookies, and potato chips, and every form of chocolate, and good quality ice cream. I am willing to learn to eat them in reasonable amounts, but I'm not willing to do without them. If you learn to eat the proper portions, you can eat anything.

I was raised in a house with very little junk food. Did I grow up to make nutritious choices as the result? No, I grew up to be completely out of control around any high fat, high sugar food product, because I'd never been taught to eat it in appropriate amounts.

Learning to eat properly has given me the tools to be in control. Learning to eat properly has given me a fighting chance to maintain a normal weight in a world that is making everyone fat.

chapter 6

Nutrition 101

Before you read any further, it's a good idea to decide why you're unhappy with your present weight. You need to question why you want to change your weight in order to determine what adjustments you're willing to make in your present diet. You have to decide not only what you want, but also why you want it. You've decided how much you want to weigh. What does that weight represent? Do you want to be a normal weight or do you want to be healthy?

It's possible to be a normal weight without being healthy; it's possible to be healthy without being a normal weight. Our family did more than just lose weight. We made changes in our eating habits and our lives that made us thinner and healthier.

It's possible to maintain a weight of 135 pounds by eating little chocolate doughnuts. As long as you consume no more than 1,600 calories per day, a little chocolate doughnut diet will maintain a weight of 135 pounds. But it won't be a good diet. It won't be a healthy diet.

In order to be healthy, our diets have to include the micronutrients: the vitamins and minerals, as well as appropriate amounts of the calorie containing macronutrients: the carbohydrates, proteins and fats. If we are to become thinner and healthier, we need to make good food choices. We need to spend some time reviewing the basics of good nutrition. Let's start with the macronutrients.

Carbohydrates

So, what exactly is a carbohydrate? When you hear the word carbohydrate, think plant. Carbohydrates are products that are directly or indirectly derived from plants. Sugars, starches, fibers and grains are all carbohydrates.

Carbohydrates 101

Carbohydrates are composed of three elements: carbon, hydrogen and oxygen. These three elements combine in a variety of forms to produce three different categories of carbohydrates: monosaccharides, disaccharides and polysaccharides.

Monosaccharides. The basic carbohydrates are the monosaccharides, the simple sugars. There are three monosaccharides. Glucose and fructose are found in fruits, vegetables, corn syrup and honey. Galactose is created when milk sugar is digested. All carbohydrates break down into some combination of glucose, fructose and galactose. The liver converts both fructose and galactose into glucose. Glucose is used directly by the cells for energy and is the body's energy currency.

Disaccharides. The second classification of carbohydrates is the disaccharides, the double sugars. The best-known sugar — sucrose — is a disaccharide. It occurs in cane, beet and maple sugar. Sucrose decomposes into a single fructose and a single glucose. Maltose, familiar to beer drinkers as malted barley, and lactose, milk sugar, are the other disaccharides. Maltose decomposes to a glucose and a glucose. Lactose decomposes into a galactose and a glucose.

Polysaccharides. The third classification of carbohydrates is the polysaccharides, commonly referred to as the complex carbohydrates, which may be composed of thousands of long strands of simple sugars. This long-strand structure allows the complex carbohydrate to be broken down slowly, providing energy in a time-released form. These complex carbohydrates may be starches or fibers. Starches include the cereal grains: wheat, rice and corn; legumes: peas and beans; and root vegetables: carrots and potatoes.

Fiber is found in plants, particularly vegetables, fruits, whole grains, nuts and legumes (beans and peas). Fiber is cellulose and cannot be digested. It may be either soluble or insoluble. Soluble fiber, which is found in oatmeal, oat bran, fruits, vegetables and legumes, assists with normal digestion, and reduces blood cholesterol levels. Insoluble fiber, commonly known as roughage, includes the skins, husks and peels of seeds, fruits and vegetables. Insoluble fiber aids in digestion by reducing the occurrence of constipation, and may help protect against colorectal cancer.

There are also indications that fiber may help to reduce blood pressure levels. In addition to these specific health benefits, the presence of fiber in diets adds bulk and helps satiate us after a meal. Unlike cows, rabbits and horses, our bodies lack the enzymes necessary to break fiber down into a usable form. As a result, we derive negligible calories from the fiber we consume.

Simple versus Complex Carbohydrates

There is tremendous confusion regarding the difference between simple carbohydrates and complex carbohydrates. Any carbohydrate that is not a simple or double sugar is a complex carbohydrate. White rice, brown rice, white flour and whole wheat flour are all complex carbohydrates. White rice and white flour are simply more processed than brown rice and whole wheat flour.

Whole grains contain all three parts of the grain kernel: the bran, the endosperm and the germ. During the milling process, the fiber and B vitamin packed bran and germ are removed, leaving only the endosperm behind. When the germ of the grain is removed, the grain becomes less nutritious, but it's still a complex carbohydrate.

In addition to grain products, fruits and vegetables are also primarily complex carbohydrates.

Why do we need carbohydrates?

Carbohydrates are the main source of our body's preferred form of energy: glucose. Glucose is the primary energy source of the central nervous system; the brain cannot survive without blood glucose, so carbohydrates are brain food. Carbohydrates are an energy source which provides approximately four calories of energy per gram of weight when converted into glucose.

Proteins

Exactly what is a protein? Proteins may originate from either plant or animal sources. Foods that contain proteins are frequently classified as combination foods because they contain more than one type of macronutrient. Proteins and fats are frequently found in combination, and meat and dairy products are the primary source combination foods that contain both protein and fat.

Proteins 101

Proteins are polymers of amino acids. Amino acids are molecules that contain one nitrogen (amino) group and one acid group (carbon, hydrogen and oxygen.) Chains of amino acids can form an almost limitless number of proteins. It is estimated that there are more than 100,000 proteins functioning in the human body.

When proteins are ingested, they are metabolized to form amino acids. Twenty different amino acids exist in food and in our bodies. Our bodies can synthesize eleven of these amino acids. The remaining nine amino acids, known as the essential amino acids, must be supplied by our diet.

The proteins that originate from animal sources are known as complete proteins, because these proteins contain all the essential amino acids. Eggs, milk, cheese, meat, poultry and fish contain complete proteins. The proteins derived from most plant sources, however, are incomplete proteins; proteins that do not provide all of the essential amino acids. Cereals, legumes, nuts and vegetable proteins are incomplete proteins. Complementary proteins are incomplete plant proteins that combine to produce all essential amino acids. Rice and beans are a classic example of a complementary protein relationship. The action of complementary proteins is particularly important to vegetarians whose diet can be protein-deficient.

Ingestion of complete or complementary proteins is key to maintaining health. Your body is continually synthesizing proteins. If a specific amino acid needed to construct a particular protein is not available, the protein will not be made. There are no substitutions for essential amino acids. If a diet is lacking a specific amino acid, the function of every protein in the body that contains that amino acid will be affected.

Why do we need protein?

Protein is responsible for all body tissue growth, repair and maintenance. The body's hormones and enzymes, as well as the antibodies our immune system uses to fight disease, are proteins. Proteins play a vital role in the structure of all body cells, in the regulation of body processes, and when our glucose stores run low, provide an alternative source of energy. The muscles in our bodies account for more than half the body's protein, and protein is normally contained in every tissue and fluid in the body with the exception of bile and urine.

The body has a very limited capacity to store amino acids. Once proteins are metabolized to amino acids, any excess amino acids are either converted to glucose, and stored as glycogen in the muscles or the liver, or converted directly to fat.

Like carbohydrates, proteins are an energy source that provides approximately four calories of energy per gram of weight.

Fats

What exactly is a fat? Fats are probably the macronutrient that receives the most attention. Most of us can identify margarine, butter, shortening and oils as types of fat. We may be less familiar, however, with the presence of fat in combination foods. The fat content in meats accounts for a significant portion of the dietary fat in the typical American diet.

Fats 101

Fat or fatty acids. Fat, or fatty acids, are the building blocks of all fats, and these fatty acids are composed of chains of carbon and hydrogen with a carboxyl (COOH) group at one end and a methyl (CH_3) group at the other end. These chains combine to form a variety of fats which may be either saturated or unsaturated.

Saturated fat. Saturated fats, such as butter or lard, are solid at room temperature, and are usually associated with animal foods. Dietary recommendations suggest that no more than one-third of the fat in our diet come from saturated fat. Since much of the fat we consume is a component of the proteins we eat, reducing the fat in our diet can be complicated. Eggs, cheese, cream, bacon, chicken and beef all contain saturated fats.

Unsaturated fat. Unsaturated fats tend to be derived from plant matter and are often liquid at room temperature. Vegetable oils such as corn, peanut and safflower, as well as avocados, hazelnuts and almonds all contain unsaturated fat. Unsaturated fat can be further divided into monounsaturated or polyunsaturated depending on the type of bonds the unsaturated fatty acids form. We should eat no more than ten percent of each type.

Why do we need fat?

Fat is a necessary part of our diet because of the important roles it plays in our bodies. While the carbohydrates we eat are our main energy source, our body's fat in the form of adipose tissue is our built-in energy reserve. Fat is also a source of and acts as a carrier for the fat-soluble vitamins: A, E, D and K.

Good fats versus bad fats.

It would be convenient if there were easy answers about good fats vs. bad fats, but the information about fats just keeps becoming more and more complicated. Generally, the unsaturated fats from vegetable oils are considered good fats because they increase the levels of high-density lipoproteins in the blood. The monounsaturated oils, such as olive oil and canola oil, are better choices than the polyunsaturated oils. Saturated fats are considered bad fats, because they increase the levels of low-density lipoproteins in the blood. Hence the recent emphasis on cooking with vegetable oils such as olive oil or canola oil, rather than with butter.

For many years, it was assumed that any dietary fat from an animal product was less healthy than a dietary fat from a plant product. As a result, margarine and shortening were considered to be healthier choices than butter. Margarine and shortening, however, are manufactured products, created by a process known as hydrogenation. During hydrogenation, hydrogen atoms are added to normally unsaturated vegetable oil. The hardness of the resulting product varies depending on the amount of saturated fat produced. One byproduct of hydrogenation is trans fatty acids, and recent studies suggest that the effects of trans fatty acids on blood lipid (fat) levels are similar to those of saturated fat.

At the same time the trans fatty acids, which are derived from a plant product, began to receive bad reviews, the Omega-3 fatty acids, which are present in animal products, began to receive positive reviews. In 1971, Danish researchers discovered a link between the Omega-3 rich diets of Eskimos living in Greenland and their low rate of cardiovascular disease. Omega-3 fatty acids are found in deep-water fish, especially the fatty varieties like albacore tuna, herring, salmon, mackerel, sardines and anchovies, as well as some leafy vegetables, seeds and oils. Additional research suggests that this type of fatty acids may also help protect us against cancer and rheumatoid arthritis.

No matter the source of the fats in our diet, there is little argument that the typical American diet contains more fat than recommended. Most dietary guidelines suggest that no more than 30 percent of total calories should come from fat. In addition, no more than 10 percent of that 30 percent should be saturated fat.

Eucalorics

High intake of fat and cholesterol is associated with atherosclerosis (vascular disease) that may lead to heart attacks and strokes. Unsaturated fats, particularly the Omega-3 fats, may improve atherosclerosis by removing cholesterol from the walls of arteries. Eating the proper types and amounts of fats, combined with daily exercise, can improve your blood lipid profile substantially, and decrease your risk of heart disease and a stroke.

The American Heart Association, American Cancer Society, American Medical Association, as well as the federal government nutrition policies all endorse a diet that contains less than 30 percent of your calories from fat, and no more than 10 percent saturated fat.

Fats are an energy source that provides approximately nine calories of energy per gram of weight. Fats are considered energy-dense, since they contain more than twice as many calories per gram as carbohydrates or proteins.

But when we walk into a store, we don't buy a carbohydrate; we buy bread. We don't buy protein; we buy cheese. In order to translate the macronutrients into daily life, we need to look at the foods that comprise a healthy diet.

chapter 7

Making Changes

eing overweight is a symptom of improper eating habits. The more overweight you are, the more changes to your diet you need to make. But,
you have to begin somewhere. Where's a sensible place to start? The federal government issues the most basic and well-known recommendations for
nutrition and health. The United
States Department of Agriculture
(USDA) and the Department of
Health and Human Services'
(HHS) Food and Drug Admin-
istration (FDA) are the two govern-
mental agencies responsible for the
Federal nutrition policies. These
policies result in a variety of recommendations. Figure 7.1 summa-
rizes the Dietary Guidelines for
Americans issued in 2000, the government's ABC's for health.

In addition to the dietary
guidelines for Americans, the government issues the Food Pyramid
Guide, and the guidelines specify
using this graphical representa-
tion, shown in Figure 7.2, to
direct food choices.

DIETARY GUIDELINES
Aim for fitness
• Aim for a healthy weight.
• Be physically active each day.
Build a healthy base
• Let the Pyramid guide your food choices.
• Choose a variety of grains daily, especially whole grains.
• Choose a variety of fruits and vegetables daily.
• Keep food safe to eat.
Choose Sensibly
• Choose a diet that is low in saturated fat and cholesterol and moderate in total fat.
• Choose beverages and foods to moderate your intake of sugars.
• Choose and prepare foods with less salt.
• If you drink alcoholic beverages, do so in moderation.

Figure 7.1

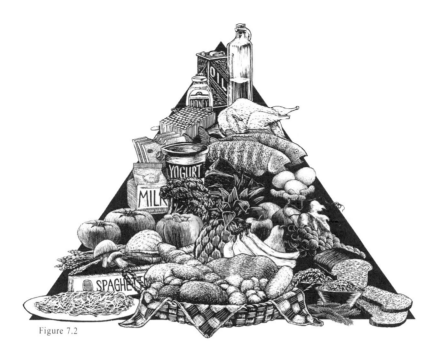

Figure 7.2

There is constant debate surrounding these seemingly innocuous and sensible guidelines. The original guidelines were issued in 1980, and new guidelines are issued every five years. This set is, therefore, the fifth set issued.

Controversy centers on the conflict between promoting health or promoting business that any adjustment in nutrition policy inevitably produces. There is intense lobbying and pressure from special interest groups, and critics maintain that these groups have detrimentally influenced the specific wording of the dietary guidelines.

I'm prepared to let the professionals argue about the nuances of word choice. I'm willing to concede that these dietary guidelines are not perfect. It's hard for me to believe, however, that the average American diet would not be significantly improved by following these admittedly imperfect guidelines.

Diane and I are not, and do not pretend to be, registered dietitians or nutrition professionals. And although Brett can certainly provide medical opinions and explanations, I decided that many of our decisions regarding nutrition require more common sense than academic training. Having been morbidly obese qualifies Diane and I to address some of the "get real" aspects of the present American diet and make sensible recommendations to change it.

In some ways, not being a professional makes it easier. I don't have to give the professional line or politically correct answer. I can hand out the "give me a break" answer. I'm not obligated to tell you what you should do; I'm allowed to acknowledge what you're going to do. I don't have to encourage perfect choices; I can get excited about proper choices. I live in the real world, not in an ivy-covered tower.

The professionals are arguing about insufficient emphasis being placed on the benefits of eating brown rice rather than refined white rice. Excuse me, please. The average fat person is eating fried rice.

They don't want me to eat a plain baked potato with chili on it because potatoes have a high glycemic index? Haven't they noticed that I'm surrounded by people eating super-sized orders of fries?

Would we be better off eating whole grain bread products? Certainly. And if we are in the process of fine-tuning an already excellent diet, than whole grains are not only the best choice, they're also a remotely possible choice. But if today's typical breakfast is biscuits with sausage gravy and hash browns, isn't hoping for whole grain toast with soy butter a tad optimistic?

Just as I believe that losing weight by subsisting on starvation rations is doomed to failure, I have similar reservations about making sudden and drastic changes in our present diets. Macrobiotic diets should probably be shelved next to fantasy weights. When we're picking out unreasonably low numbers for our scales, we're contemplating food choices we normally wouldn't feed the hamster. If your present diet is a veritable banquet of high fat, high sugar choices, don't decide to go cold turkey on junk food on the first day. It's easier and less stressful to make gradual changes to your diet. If you've been a fast food aficionado, now is not the time for heroic changes. Start by adding fruits and vegetables to your diet. You can always add bulgur and tofu later.

My previous diet was not a healthy diet, and there's a good chance that your present diet looks like my old diet. There is a reason we are doing so poorly. Surveys about diets indicate that most people are overwhelmed by the amount of information available. As a result of the epidemic of obesity, the media gives significant airtime to issues concerning overweight and obesity, but today's message may not agree with yesterday's message. And confident, well-spoken individuals with impressive letters after their name delivered both messages. How do we decide who to believe?

Start with the basics. Let's take a look at the food pyramid and use the common sense approach to dietary choices. Most of us know what we're supposed to be doing; we're just not doing it. Do it one category at a time. Do what looks reasonable. If one set of recommendations clearly isn't going to happen in your life, don't throw up your hands in frustration and walk away from the entire list. Do what seems possible.

Grains

The base of the pyramid creates instant guilt. The minute I read whole grain, I start to feel like the world's worst mother, because my children don't eat whole grain bread products. And my children are not alone. We're all eating lots of grains, but we're eating them in highly processed, high fat, high sugar and high calorie snack food. We're supposed to be eating whole grains and we're eating doughnuts. And the distance between those two choices appears insurmountable.

Most of the reason we are told to eat whole grains is for the fiber. If whole grain bread and brown rice aren't in your future, what about eating more fruits and vegetables? If you eat your fruits and vegetables, you'll get lots of fiber, and you won't have to feel as guilty about eating white bread. Do what you can. The goal is to improve.

Want some good news? Popcorn is considered a whole grain product. I buy the 94 percent fat-free microwave popcorn and I often eat it as my evening snack. Oatmeal is a whole grain. I eat lots of oatmeal. I'm even thinking about eating brown rice. Diane is not.

Fruit

The goal is two fruits per day, a variety of fruit and whole fruit rather than fruit juice. How are we doing? We're not eating enough, and five fruits account for nearly half the fruit consumption in this country and two of those are juices: orange juice, bananas, fresh apples, watermelon and apple juice. How do we improve? We need to eat more fruit, and we should aim for variety. Since most of us like fruit, it's not hard to add fruit to our diet. It makes a good morning or afternoon snack. Or start substituting fruit for those heavy and fattening desserts.

Vegetables

You probably remember vegetables. They're the category of food we're all supposed to eat that we don't. In my previous life, my attitude toward vegetables was simple. I didn't eat them. I ate salads, but the greens were drowning in full-fat dressing. I ate potatoes, but the potato was loaded with butter, sour cream and bacon. Now I eat vegetables. I may be doing crummy with whole grains, but I eat lots of vegetables. I eat asparagus and sugar snap peas; I eat stewed tomatoes and okra; I eat broccoli and cauliflower. I am totally and completely amazed at what I eat.

Give vegetables a chance. Remind yourself that Diane and I didn't eat vegetables before and now we do. Look at our pictures and consider the possibility that vegetables are responsible for this amazing transformation. You've been willing to try almost anything to lose weight, haven't you? How bad could eating a few vegetables be compared to some of the things you've tried?

Here are the rules:
- If it's fried, it doesn't count as a vegetable.
- If it's covered with cheese, it doesn't count as a vegetable.
- If it's swimming in a cream sauce, it doesn't count as a vegetable.
- Potatoes, corn and peas count as starches, not vegetables.

What's left? Look at the menus. Every dinner has a vegetable. Remember the three hundred pounds? Give vegetables a chance. I started by adding peeled baby carrots as an afternoon snack. They come in a small package, don't need to be washed, don't require a utensil and don't need to be cooked. Pretend they're not good for you and it should be easy to add them to your diet.

Milk Products

This one is easy. Drink and eat the low fat and skim versions of these products. If you normally drink whole milk, start drinking two percent. If you normally drink two percent, start drinking one percent. If you normally drink one percent, start drinking skim. Drink a lower fat version for three weeks or four weeks. Chose the next lower fat product and repeat the process until you're drinking skim. I mixed one percent and skim for three weeks.

Don't whine about it. Nobody likes to listen to a whiner. Just ask Diane. (Yeah, I did a lot of whining about skim milk.)

Why drink skim milk? Why eat low-fat sour cream and cottage cheese? Fewer calories. Less fat.

Meat, Poultry, Fish and Seafood

Most Americans get their protein from beef, veal, pork and lamb. According to the Center for Science in the Public Interest (CSPI), 45 percent of the beef sold in the US is ground beef. Have we given up beef? No. We eat ground beef and include recipes that use ground beef in this book. But we only use the lowest fat version of ground beef available: extra-lean ground beef.

We also eat a great deal of pork, but we only use the leanest cut of pork available, the center cut of the pork loin. Or pork tenderloins.

Why use the lower-fat beef and pork products? Fewer calories. Less fat.

We eat lots of chicken; the recipes in the book use boneless, skinless chicken breasts. We also eat fish and seafood. Chicken, fish and seafood are naturally lower in fat, especially saturated fat, than red meat products.

If you're struggling with being overweight and have spent your life eating "meat and potatoes," now might be a good time to consider expanding your culinary horizons.

Fat and Oils

Fat and oils share the tip of the Food Pyramid with sweets. The fat in our diets comes not only from fats and oils, but also from the fat in meat and diary products. If we are not careful, fat sneaks into our diets. Many foods are combination foods; they are single foods that contain more than one macronutrient. Most people think of dairy products as protein, but full fat dairy products are often fats masquerading as protein. Choose full fat milk, cottage cheese, sour cream and yogurt rather than the low fat versions of the same product, and you're getting lots of fat with your protein.

Cheddar cheese is America's favorite cheese, and it accounts for 65 percent of cheese consumption. It's also a protein whose calorie content more closely resembles a fat; it contains, in addition to seven grams of protein, a staggering nine grams of fat per ounce.

Cheese is not the only fat that masquerades as a protein. Meats such as bacon and sausage contain, gram for gram, more fat than protein. Even a plant based protein source, such as peanut butter, can provide more fat than protein in a serving.

Salad dressings are another source of fat and calories. The average woman frequently chooses salads as a low calorie alternative to a sandwich, but a study found that women aged 19-50 get more fat in their diet from salad dressing, than any other food source.

Switch to the low fat and skim versions of dairy products and the extra lean versions of beef and pork, and you'll not only reduce your diet's caloric content, but you'll also greatly reduce its fat content. Start getting your salad dressing on the side and you'll be in even better shape.

Sweets

We're all eating lots of sugar. Our consumption of snack foods has not only reduced our consumption of fiber and complex carbohydrates, but also has helped skyrocket our consumption of added sugar. Sugar consumption in the United States has risen 28 percent since 1983.

The government suggests we get no more than the equivalent of ten teaspoons of sugar, if we are eating a healthy diet of 2,000 calories. The average American is consuming sugar at a rate three times the recommended amount, one quarter of a pound per day.

Where is the sugar in food located? It's in the highly processed foods. In 1909, two-thirds of the sugar produced was used in the home. Today, three-quarters of the sugar produced is used commercially. It's listed by a variety of different names on food labels and shows up on our waistlines as added sugar in soda, cakes, cookies and candy.

Why should you care about added sugar? In a word — calories. Sugar supplies calories without nutrients and fiber. It is instant energy that the body doesn't have to do any work to get. If you have a limited number of calories, sugar displaces healthier alternatives.

As I lost weight, I made significant changes in my eating habits. My present diet bears little resemblance to my previous diet and I am continually amazed at the transformation that has occurred. This revolution in eating habits occurred gradually and I would never have believed it was possible to make this dramatic a change in my eating habits at this point in my life. But it was.

In order for me to be mentally and physically happy with my daily caloric allotment, I have made permanent changes in my eating habits. Do I eat perfectly? No. But, I consistently make better food choices. My head and my body are happy with my present diet.

chapter 8

The Big Bad World of Food

Y ou've learned a little nutrition. You recognize the Food Pyramid. You're ready to make some changes to your imperfect diet. Out the door you go, into the real world. A world filled with food.

Food is everywhere. Walk the aisles at the grocery store on a Saturday afternoon and it's possible to consume a meal's worth of calories. They pass out samples: a new variety of cookie, a slice of deli cheese on a cracker, a little piece of pizza, a taste of cheesecake. And it's not just the grocery store. There are chocolate coins at the bank, mints by the restaurant cashier and toffees at the dry cleaners.

The United States food industry is presently producing 3,800 calories per day for each and every man, woman and child in America. After adjusting for wasted calories, such as leftovers, spoilage and oil used for frying, that number becomes 2,680 calories per day.

What happens if you're female and you consistently consume your share of this abundance of available food? If the food supply creates 2,680 calories a day just for you, and you eat it, what will you weigh based on the 12 calories per pound calculation?

$$\frac{2{,}680 \text{ calories}}{12 \text{ calories/pound}} = 223 \text{ pounds}$$

What if you're male?

$$\frac{2,680 \text{ calories}}{14 \text{ calories/pound}} = 191 \text{ pounds}$$

Where do all these calories go? To our hips, to our thighs, to our waists. What's the inevitable result of this abundance of calories? We're all fat. We're all fat because we're surrounded by food. All day. All the time. Everywhere we go. Specifically, we're surrounded by junk food.

Junk Food

What is junk food? It's the high sugar, high sodium, high calorie food that provides little or no nutrition. It's eaten while standing or driving; it's eaten when bored or upset. It's eaten without regard to the calories it contains. It's the readily available, rapidly consumed and quickly forgotten food that packs amazing amounts of calories in remarkably small packages. There is calorie and nutritional information on each and every bag of chips and bar of chocolate, but it could be printed in hieroglyphics for all the attention it receives.

While our minds are ignoring the calories that junk food contains, our waistlines and hips are paying attention. And junk food is available anywhere you go. It's at the checkout line in every conceivable type of store. Whether you're purchasing copier paper, or a hammer, or three yards of lace, you can walk away from the cash register with chocolate in your chubby little fist.

Junk food is easy to eat. It doesn't need to be washed; it doesn't need to be peeled or chopped. It doesn't require a knife or fork, pots and pans, an oven or a microwave. It's quickly transformed from potential calories in a package to extra inches on your thighs, and this transformation is occurring every day, everywhere, to everyone. As a result of this omnipresent banquet of junk food, an increasing percentage of our daily caloric intake is devoted to fat and sugar.

The macronutrients, the carbohydrates, proteins and fats are calorie-containing sources of energy. Carbohydrates and proteins provide four calories of energy per gram of food; fats provide nine calories of energy per gram of food. Fats are, therefore, considered to be energy dense foods. Lots of calories packed in small packages.

In order for our bodies to be happy with the caloric intake that maintains a normal weight, we need to be smart calorie consumers. We are all smart shoppers. We look for sales. We search out bargains. We recognize the value of the good deal. We need to apply our sharply honed shopping skills to the world of food. We need to start recognizing the good deal foods. These are the foods that maximize the amount of food we can eat without maximizing the number of calories we're consuming.

Fats are expensive calories. Lots of calories without much food volume. And the less food we consume, the less likely that our body will feel full and satisfied within the caloric window that supports our normal weight.

Food Preparation

Studies indicate that we base the amount we eat on the volume of food we consume. It takes a certain amount of food to feel full. Our bodies aren't running a tape on the calories we're consuming; our bodies are running a tape on the volume we're consuming. It's possible to eat a significantly larger volume of food by making smart calorie consumer food and preparation choices. Let's look at an example.

Start with a high fiber, low calorie, complex carbohydrate: the potato.

An ordinary baking potato with skin has approximately 20 calories and 0 grams of fat per ounce.

Now, cut that same potato into six wedges, introduce them to a deep fat fryer, and suddenly the baked potato becomes cottage fries that have 70 calories and four grams of fat per ounce. If you prefer thin fries, it's easy to reach 90 calories and five grams of fat per ounce. Slice the potato paper thin, and the all-American potato chip arrives at 150 calories and 10 grams of fat per ounce.

Variations in food preparation have increased the potato's calories per ounce data, from 20 calories per ounce to 150 calories per ounce.

What about energy density? What effect did preparation have on the potatoes energy density?

Baked Potato:

$$\frac{20 \text{ calories/ounce}}{28 \text{ grams/ounce}} = 0.71 \text{ calories/gram}$$

Potato Chips:

$$\frac{150 \text{ calories/ounce}}{28 \text{ grams/ounce}} = 5.36 \text{ calories/gram}$$

The plain baking potato has an energy density of .71; our potato chips have an energy density of 5.36. The energy density of the chips is nearly seven and a half times as large as the energy density of the baking potato.

Why should you care?

It means that you can eat seven and a half times as much baked potato as potato chips for the same number of calories. Eating low energy density food means you can eat enough food to feel full until your next meal. Eating low energy density food means maintaining weight loss by making long-term changes in the way you eat.

Complex carbohydrates, particularly fruits and vegetables, have low energy densities. Steamed rice and naked pasta are good food choice carbohydrates. Take those same foods and fry them, cover them with butter and a cream sauce, and good choices become bad choices.

Nearly 70 percent of the added fat in our diet comes from salad oil, cooking oil and shortening. Plus, the average American is still consuming more than 34 percent of their calories from fat. As long as we continue to eat french fries and potato chips, especially in larger and larger portions, we're not making good food choices.

High sugar, high fat, highly processed foods are generally very energy dense foods. It is estimated that 20 percent of the calories we consume are coming from cakes, cookies, pies, pastries, ice cream, pudding, sugar, candy, syrup, soda, non-carbonated beverages, corn chips, tortilla chips and potato chips. The consumption of high fat, high sugar snack foods doubled between 1977 and 1994.

If I can only eat 1,600 calories a day, I want those to be the best tasting, most flavorful calories I can find. Highly processed foods contain sugar, salt, fat, and natural and artificial flavorings that are added to compensate for the nutrients and flavor removed by the processing procedures. Low nutrition, low fiber, processed foods provide expensive calories that do not make my body happy with the volume of food it has received. But, it is particularly difficult to avoid snacking in today's world.

Does it make that much difference? It can. It is very easy to add 200-300 calories to your day by consuming a single candy bar. I picked up a chocolate bar at the grocery store yesterday to look at the nutritional information. My favorite candy bar would add a quick 280 calories to my caloric intake. If I'm already consuming the amount of calories that I'm balancing by physical activity, what does this do to my weight?

$$3{,}500 \text{ calories/pound} / 280 \text{ calories/ day} = 12.5 \text{ days to gain a pound}$$

$$365 \text{ days/year} / 12.5 \text{ days/pound} = 29 \text{ pounds/year}$$

I haven't allowed any calories for digestion, so that number is not completely accurate, but it's still a pretty scary number. It demonstrates that it doesn't take very many extra calories to gain weight.

If you've become fairly casual about picking up a little something to tide you over until dinner, and you don't adjust dinner to compensate for those extra calories, snacking could be one explanation for some of your weight problems. If you're a tall male who can eat 2,600 calories a day, it's easier to find calories for snacking. And it's not as critical for those snacks to be nutritious. If you're a petite female, you don't have many extra calories to spare. If you want to be the correct weight, and eat a healthy diet, it's difficult to find room for junk food.

The Month of Candy Madness

My previous diet was filled with junk food. And it wasn't easy to give it up at first. The first Halloween after we started dieting was October 2000. We had been dieting for approximately four months when the snack sized candy bars appeared at the grocery store. Each bar contained about 50 calories. An easy and attractive size for a snack. We bought a bag.

We were initially very pleased with ourselves. We carefully noted the calories consumed each day in chocolate. We never binged. We were doing so well, it seemed safe to have more than one kind available, so we bought another bag. We never exceeded our daily caloric allotment, but the number of calories assigned to chocolate kept getting bigger. And neither one of us wanted to admit what was happening. Eventually, I was up to 400 calories in chocolate, 25 percent of my daily calories. And I was hungry, because the energy-dense chocolate didn't provide enough food for the calories it contained.

We dubbed it, The Month of Candy Madness, and it hasn't been repeated. It was our first lesson in the power of energy density, and it gave birth to the concept of the saturation of the senses. To the idea that the first bite tastes best.

Saturation of the Senses

There is medical evidence that all senses become saturated. Smells are strongest when first detected. Water feels hottest at the first touch. Does excessive eating also saturate our taste buds? If it does, then the first bite actually does taste best. If the product is not wonderful, it will not improve by continued consumption. If we keep eating until the bag is empty, all we will accomplish is emptying the bag. If the first bite doesn't provide the proper level of mouth pleasure, we'll never get it by consuming more.

Some of the best tasting food is served as hors d'oeuvres; single bites of intense flavors. Tasting menus provide small portions of multiple courses. Expensive wines are sampled by swirling a single taste in the mouth. All of these examples could lend credence to the unnoticed fact that the first bite tastes best.

Perhaps overeating is an unconscious effort to recreate the intense flavor associated with that first mouth-watering bite. If you eat only the best food you can, and you pay attention to what you eat, and you savor every bite, it's much easier to be satisfied with the proper portions of food.

It's hard, however, to be selective when we are surrounded by food prepared by others. As more and more food is consumed away from home, we have slowly relinquished a large portion of control over the food we consume. And the result has been an epidemic of obesity. If we've all been participants in an eating experiment, it's time to decide that the experiment has failed.

How can you exist in this world of caloric abundance and maintain a normal weight? You're taking the first step. The first step is recognizing the cause and the extent of the problem. Once you acknowledge the severity of the problem, you can start learning to co-exist with this ubiquitous supply of food. In order to control how much food you're eating, you have to pay attention. You have to play an active role in deciding what goes in your mouth.

Learning to eat properly is not a spectator sport!

The number of overweight and obese people continue to spiral upward, because the world in which we live makes it easy to be fat and difficult to be thin. It's easier to lose and maintain weight by learning to eat properly, instead of dieting, but being a normal weight still requires self-discipline.

Thin Women Don't Eat Quiche

I'd spent most of my life convinced that thin women were different. It was easy to believe that thin women were genetically blessed. I was sure they ate anything and everything they wanted and didn't gain weight. Or perhaps they were allergic to chocolate and didn't like the taste of ice cream.

The truth? There are a few women who are genetically blessed. But not many. Most women who are a normal weight are no more genetically blessed than you and I. They are thin because they have decided to be thin. They are thin because they work at it. The athletic clubs are filled with thin women sweating on treadmills and cross-trainers and watching every morsel they pop in their mouths. The woman who looks great in her jeans very likely walks, runs, plays tennis or spends time on a Nordic track or an elliptical trainer. Her chicken is grilled and her dressing is ALWAYS, ALWAYS, ALWAYS eaten on the side.

Talk to the women at the gym. Why are they there? They're there so they can eat more food. Fat and sugar taste good. And if you eat them in the proper portions, there is no reason that you cannot continue to eat them. But you can't eat as much as you want. As much as you have been. You can't eat them all the time.

Have I given up candy bars? No. But, I don't pick one up casually. When I do decide to eat one, I make sure I enjoy every bite I put in my mouth. I can afford the calories for an occasional candy bar, but I can't calorically afford to eat bags or boxes or pints of high fat, high sugar junk food. So I don't.

When I eat an energy dense food, I make sure it's worth the calories it contains. I'm perfectly willing to spend calories on excellent quality food. I'm no longer willing to waste the calories that maintain a normal weight on mediocre food.

chapter 9

High Maintenance Eating

I read lots of books on dieting, and I was fascinated by the books that told me to listen to my body to know when I was full. My amused reaction was, Excuse me? You obviously haven't noticed that I'm 100 pounds overweight (Okay, okay, maybe 120). If I knew when my body was full, I wouldn't be in this shape. I didn't rely on internal signals to tell me when I was finished eating. I relied on external signals.

When are we finished eating? When the bag is empty. When our plate is clean. When the cupboard is bare. When are we finished eating? We're finished when the food is gone.

If you are tremendously overweight, you have been abusing your body for years; your stomach no longer sends the appropriate "I'm full" signals. The goal is to be able to listen to your body. But, first, your body needs help. Your body needs to be consistently fed properly until your body learns how much food you should be eating. Your body needs to be taught how a proper portion of food looks and tastes.

But, food portions are not one size fits all. The more calories it takes to support a normal weight, the more servings or larger portions that can be consumed. Men have a higher calorie factor (14 instead of 12) than women. This differential in the calorie factor means that it is more difficult for the average woman to achieve and maintain a normal weight than it is for the average man, because she can eat fewer calories.

If you're a female with a goal weight of 150 pounds, it takes 1,800 calories per day to maintain that weight. If you're a male, it takes 2,100 calories to maintain the same goal weight of 150 pounds. The man has a caloric advantage of three hundred calories per day. Where does this advantage come from?

Muscle mass. Men's bodies average 22 percent muscle; women's bodies average 15 percent muscle. Even if a woman and a man are the same height and the same weight, the man gets to eat more food to sustain that weight than the woman due to his increased muscle mass. Muscle burns more calories than fat, so the natural tendency of men to have a higher muscle mass means they can eat more calories than a woman of identical height and weight.

The average man is also taller than the average woman. Since height is one of the factors in the BMI calculation, the average man can weigh more than the average woman due to his increased height and still have a normal weight as defined by the BMI calculations.

The realities of weight are particularly harsh for someone like me. I'm a 5'2" female. With whom shall I register my complaint? My mother who is 5' tall or my grandfather who was 5'4"? When I sit down to dinner with just about anyone, male or female, they're going to get to eat more than I do. If you're female, it's particularly hard to be thin. If you're a short female, it's even harder. You simply don't have very many extra calories to play with.

Remember the definition of proper eating? Consuming a nutritious, well-balanced, variety of foods in the proper portions to maintain a normal weight. The goal of a diet is weight loss. The goal of proper eating is health. A normal weight is one aspect of health, but it is only one. If you're a female, it's easier to focus on being healthy than on being thin. Focus on eating properly and don't obsess about your weight. But you need to start by acknowledging that your extra weight has been the result of eating extra calories. How many extra calories?

Take another look at the number of calories that will support your goal weight, then calculate how many calories you've been eating to support your present weight. How many extra calories are you presently consuming? We'll use my numbers as an example.

247 pounds x 12 = 2,964 calories
135 pounds x 12 = 1,620 calories
2964-1620 = 1,344 calories

Fill in your numbers below.

Present weight:

_____ x 12 (women) = _____
x 14 (men)

Goal weight:

_____ x 12 (women) = _____
x 14 (men)

Excess calories:

_____ - _____ = _____
Present calories   **Goal Calories**   **Excess Calories**

What did those 1,344 extra calories represent? Easily available calories. When I paid no attention to making good food choices, food preparation or to caloric content, I averaged 2,964 calories per day, and 1,344 of those calories were the difference between being morbidly obese and being a normal weight.

The heavier you are, the more extra calories you're consuming. If most of your meals are eaten away from home, a significant number of those extra calories are the result of unreasonable portion sizes. When we eat out, we relinquish control. And, in the modern world of meals outside the home, a variety of complex social and economic factors influences the meals and portions we receive.

If you're trying to be healthy while eating out, there are usually about three choices on the menu that appear remotely possible. One of them is grilled chicken, and the other two sound nasty. You order the grilled chicken and a salad, and you end up feeling sorry for yourself. The next thing you know, you're having the chocolate brownie á la mode to make yourself feel better.

How big should a portion be? How many calories should it contain? It depends. Who's going to eat this meal? Short, inactive, older females should be consuming smaller amounts of food, than growing adolescent males. The caloric intake should be a function of height, weight and activity level of the diner. In the restaurant business, however, these decisions are based on economic considerations.

How do we get you into our restaurant? How do we maximize the amount of money you will spend? And, how do we get you to come back? Unfortunately, the answer to all three questions has been identical. More food. The perception of value, of "getting your money's worth," is based on larger and larger portions of food.

The fast food industry should be credited with the invention of the instantaneously variable portion size. Since the object was to increase the average check, however, the variability only went one way — up. The industry started with combination meals whose initial appeal was based on ordering convenience and savings. Order a sandwich, fries and a drink and pay less than ordering the components individually. The combination meals are prominently displayed, so it's easy to make a quick decision to go for the good deal.

After we were all trained to order combination meals, the next great idea was increased sizes. For a nominal increase in price, you could get more fries and a bigger drink. Now, this is a great idea. More fries. Yum-yum, fat calories to go in a convenient paper container. Since fries and soda have the highest profit margins, the majority of that 39 cents is pure profit.

Both combination meals and increased sizes are designed to maximize corporate revenue. There are 170,000 fast food restaurants in the United States, and those restaurants spend $3 billion dollars a year on advertising. When a customer arrives at a specific restaurant, it is imperative that the money spent per customer is maximized. The restaurant's overhead costs are, of course, based on a variety of expenses. Since food costs are low, consistently increasing the average sale through combination meals and increased sizes are great business decisions.

If you examine both the monetary and health costs of these selling techniques, are we, the consumer, making wise decisions while we increase the profits of the fast food industry?

Figuring the economic cost is easy. More food for the bargain price of 39 cents. What about the health ramifications? Let's start with the regular order of fries. Anybody out there know how many calories are in a typical order of French fries?

> How about 440 calories and 19 grams of fat?
> And, if you increase the size of those fries?
> A quick 530 calories and 23 grams of fat.

What about real soda? Take a look at Table 9.2.

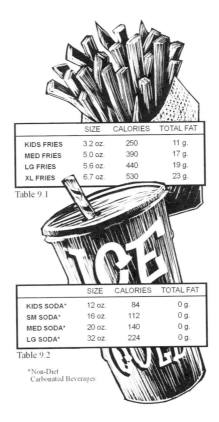

	SIZE	CALORIES	TOTAL FAT
KIDS FRIES	3.2 oz.	250	11 g.
MED FRIES	5.0 oz.	390	17 g.
LG FRIES	5.6 oz.	440	19 g.
XL FRIES	6.7 oz.	530	23 g.

Table 9.1

	SIZE	CALORIES	TOTAL FAT
KIDS SODA*	12 oz.	84	0 g.
SM SODA*	16 oz.	112	0 g.
MED SODA*	20 oz.	140	0 g.
LG SODA*	32 oz.	224	0 g.

Table 9.2

*Non-Diet
Carbonated Beverages

The presence of self-service refills encourages customers to maximize the non-nutritious sugar calories present in soft drinks. Since a higher proportion of males drink sugared soda, the high caloric content of soda is of particular concern for the overweight adolescent male population.

This information is not presented with the expectation that you'll never eat fast food again, but to emphasize the necessity of making informed choices when ordering fast food. If you're the average woman, 5'4" in height, 148 pounds in weight and eating 1,800 calories per day, an upsized order of fries represents 29 percent of your calories and 38 percent of your fat for the entire day. That's just the fries. That's before you even touch your sandwich.

Remember my own personal favorite and frequently consumed fast food meal, 1,310 calories and 45 grams of fat? Those numbers are based on diet soda. If regular soda is added, the calories increase to 1,450. Spend an extra 39 cents to up-size that meal, and 1,624 calories are accompanied by 51 artery-clogging fat grams.

Eucalorics

If you are female, eating out magnifies some of the not fair realities of life. In the unfair world of fast food, a child's meal consisting of a cheeseburger, fries, and a diet soda has 577 calories and 26 grams of fat. The average woman should be ordering a child's meal, not a combination meal.

Restaurants

The trend toward increased portion sizes is everywhere. If you sell bagels, make your bagels bigger. How much bigger? If you check a calorie guide, a bagel is listed as having 80 calories. But that's a one-ounce bagel and the average bagel may weigh three, four, or even five ounces. The bagel purchased from my favorite bagel store weighed 3.5 ounces. That's about 280 calories, and that's before you put anything on it. The problem with consistently eating that size bagel is that your stomach begins to think that 3.5 ounces of bagel, plus cream cheese, is a normal portion.

If you order lunch at just about any Chinese restaurant, you'll get about 2 cups of rice. Two cups of rice must be a serving, right? And a serving of rice has about a hundred calories. Well, you're half right. A serving of rice does have about a hundred calories, but a serving is half a cup. You've just been given four servings of rice. And that's white rice, not fried rice. How many of us are ordering white rice, if fried rice is the same price? And what becomes of proper portions at the ever-popular Chinese buffet? When a study evaluated buffet-style restaurants, it was determined that the amount of food consumed was related to the number of entrées. The more entrées, the more food each person consumed.

Everybody likes getting something for nothing, so the standard first course in many restaurants is announced by the timely arrival of chips and salsa, cheese biscuits or loaves of bread. Instant alleviation of hunger makes everyone content and more tolerant of any delays in service that may occur due to understaffing or other unavoidable problems. Unfortunately, it's easy to consume enough calories in that first free course to constitute dinner, before dinner is even ordered, much less arrives and is eaten. The cost of those chips may not show up on the dinner check, but they do show up when you step on the scales.

It's very difficult to lose weight and keep it off, if you eat most of your meals away from home. If you do eat out, you have to be particularly vigilant. You have to become a high maintenance eater.

"I'd like the Asian salad. But without the sesame noodles or the almonds, and I'd like the dressing on the side. And could you please add cucumbers and red onion?"

"I'd like the Santa Fe chicken. But I'd like the sauce on the side, and no bacon or cheese. And please make sure the breast is skinned. And I'd like a baked potato instead of fries, and the butter and the sour cream on the side."

In the movie "When Harry Met Sally," Harry Burns (Billy Crystal) says to Sally Albright (Meg Ryan), "On the side is a very big thing with you." High maintenance eating is "Dining With Sally Albright." Everything is always on the side. Is it possible to eat out and lose weight? Yes. But it requires both diligence and determination.

I previously ate lots of high fat, high sugar, highly processed food. Now I eat very little. Once I started eating the proper foods in the proper portions, I decided that many products I previously ate in excess simply weren't worth the calories. The longer I ate properly, the easier it became to discriminate between foods. And when I eat out, I'm a high maintenance patron.

chapter 10

No One's in the Kitchen with Dinah

E ating properly involves an ongoing and constant battle against the omnipresent high fat and high sugar environment in which we live and eating out magnifies those difficulties. Diane and I responded to those difficulties by starting to cook again. We believe there are basic survival skills necessary to win the battle against being overweight, and rudimentary cooking skills are high on the survival skill list. If you spend at least some time in the kitchen, you will be able to have more control over the food you eat. Plus, you'll be able to eat a wider variety of food.

As we have moved further and further away from preparing food at home, we have become fatter and fatter, and the quality of the food that we routinely consume has decreased. It is very difficult to eat well if you rely completely on others to prepare your food.

Eucalorics is easier to follow than a typical diet because it allows you to have more calories, more food. It's easier to eat sensibly when you're not hungry. How can you maximize your calories? How can you have the most control over what goes in your mouth? Cook.

Order meatloaf at a restaurant and you'll have no idea about the grade of ground beef used to prepare it. Prepare it yourself and you can choose extra-lean ground beef. Eat out, and you're going to be frustrated by the lack of healthy choices on the menu. Cook, and every meal can taste good and be healthy.

When did I become fat? When did my children become fat? When I quit cooking. I grew up surrounded by cooks. My grandmother, my mother and my aunts cooked. My childhood memories of holidays are filled with the sights and sounds and smells of wonderful food. I had always cooked without much regard to calories or fat content and had battled my weight all my life, but my weight only spiraled completely out of control when I stopped cooking. Is my family different? Not according to the statistics.

Food Away From Home

Food away from home is defined as food that is not purchased at a retail store such as a grocery store or a gas station. Food away from home includes pizza that is delivered to a private home and includes Chinese take out. The number of meals eaten away from home has increased from 13 percent in 1977 to 29 percent in 1995. The calories consumed away from home are also rising. The statistics indicate that meals in restaurants or fast food places contribute a higher percentage of calories and fat than meals eaten at home.

In the last hundred years, the effort required on the part of the consumer to produce meals has been steadily reduced. Homemade has become a style of food rather than food made at home. Fried chicken comes in a bucket. Biscuits come in cans. Teaching a child to bake cookies has been reduced to taking a premixed, preformed cookie from a package and placing it on a cookie sheet.

We kept telling people that we were losing weight because we were eating really well. But it was difficult to get anyone to believe us. No one believes that it is possible to prepare meals that are low calorie and low fat which are filling and taste good. But it is.

How did we lose so much weight? We started to cook again, but we changed the way we cooked. We began to alter our recipes and devise new ones to meet the caloric and fat requirements of our new eating regime. We ate really well, so we did not suffer the feelings of deprivation that appeared to inevitably lead to binging.

Changing the way we cooked, also involved changing the way we shopped. Most of us are in a hurry when we shop. We're tired, we're hungry and we routinely buy the same brands or what's on sale. Diane and I spent a lot of time in grocery stores. We spent a lot of time standing around reading labels and taking notes.

Nutrition Labels

In 1990, congress passed the Nutrition Labeling and Education Act (NLEA) that was enacted in 1994. This legislation requires all packaged food to carry a nutrition label. The label includes the number of servings per container, the serving size, the calories per serving, and the calories from total and saturated fat. Additional information about cholesterol, sodium, total carbohydrate, dietary fiber, sugar and protein is also included. The amounts of the vitamins A and D, and the minerals calcium and iron are listed.

Figure 10.1 provides a sample food label. Labels contain a great deal of information that can be extremely useful in counting calories and fat grams, or determining other relevant health information about a product. The presence of nutritional labels on so many food products makes counting calories and other nutrients much easier.

Nutrition Facts

Serving Size 1/2 cup dry (40g)
Servings Per Container see UPC table

Amount Per Serving

	Cereal Alone	with 1/2 cup Vitamin A&D Fortified Skim Milk
Calories	150	190
Calories from Fat	25	25

	% Daily Value*	
Total Fat 3g*	5%	5%
Saturated Fat 0.5g	2%	2%
Polyunsaturated Fat 1g		
Monounsaturated Fat 1g		
Cholesterol 0mg	0%	0%
Sodium 0mg	0%	3%
Total Carbohydrate 27g	9%	11%
Dietary Fiber 4g	15%	15%
Soluble Fiber 2g		
Insoluble Fiber 2g		
Sugars 1g		
Protein 5g		
Vitamin A	0%	4%
Vitamin C	0%	2%
Calcium	0%	15%
Iron	10%	10%

* Amount in Cereal. One half cup skim milk contributes an additional 40 Calories, 65mg Sodium, 200mg Potassium, 6g Total Carbohydrate (6g Sugars), and 4g Protein.
** Percent Daily Values are based on a 2,000 calorie diet. Your daily values may be higher or lower depending on your calorie needs:

	Calories	2,000	2,500
Total Fat	Less than	65g	80g
Sat. Fat	Less than	20g	25g
Cholesterol	Less than	300mg	300mg
Sodium	Less than	2,400mg	2,400mg
Total Carbohydrate		300g	375g
Dietary Fiber		25g	30g

Calories per gram:
Fat 9 · Carbohydrate 4 · Protein 4

Figure 10.1 Food Label

Labels are only useful, however, if you pay attention. The information of a label is based on serving size. If you eat an *entire* muffin whose calorie and fat information is based on a serving size of *half* a muffin, you have just eaten twice as many calories as you thought. If a product is some type of a mix, the nutritional information is for the mix alone. It is optional to include the nutritional information of the prepared product.

Diane and I purchased a scone mix that listed its calorie content as 110 calories per scone. But, that number was based only on the contents of the mix. Add milk, eggs and 12 tablespoons of butter, and the calorie content of the final product is frighteningly different than the number on the box.

Making Good Product Choices

If you are careful, food labels can be a powerful tool to help improve your diet. One of the most useful ways to use the information on food labels is to compare similar products. We cook Mexican food, so we stood in the aisle of the grocery store and compared tortillas. In addition to variations from brand to brand, there are size variations within a brand. The Kroger grocery chain carries three different sizes just in their store brand.

	CALORIES	FAT GRAMS
Kroger, fajita:	80	0.5
Kroger, taco:	150	4.0
Kroger, burrito	220	5.0
Old El Paso, taco	80	2.25
Aztec, taco	130	2.5
Mission, burrito	220	5.0

Table 10.1

Now, a tortilla is basically a neutral starch used to wrap around other food. So, why not choose the tortilla with the lowest calorie and least amount of fat? What's the big deal?

Remember the discussions about portion sizes? We've trained ourselves to routinely consume portions that are too large. We need to learn to eat smaller portions. If two tacos are a normal serving of tacos, reducing the calories in the tacos by using a fajita size tortilla instead of a taco size tortilla reduces the calories in the tortillas by 140 calories and 8.0 grams of fat.

But it also takes less meat and cheese to fill the smaller tortilla. Perhaps rather than three ounces of meat per taco, you use two ounces of meat, and one ounce of cheese, instead of two. That saves approximately 100 calories and three grams of fat in meat, and 110 calories and nine grams of fat in cheese. For a total difference of 350 calories and 20 grams of fat. If you eat tacos twice a month for a year, that savings is equal to the calories in about two pounds.

A main course for dinner that consists of two tortillas, four ounces of meat, one ounce of cheese, lettuce and tomato, equals 470 calories and 15 grams of fat. This meal meets the government recommendations of no more than 30 percent of calories from fat.

The most important factor is that eating smaller tacos is a better choice than not eating tacos at all. The fastest way to start feeling deprived is to start treating any food as forbidden or illegal. We made adjustments in our recipes and our portion sizes, so we could eat everything. We didn't feel deprived, so we didn't binge. We lost the weight we wanted to lose and we have kept the weight off.

Similar variations exist in every other product. Bread varies from 40 calories and .25 grams of fat per slice for light to 150 calories and two grams of fat per slice for regular. Again, is it a big deal? Over a lifetime of bread consumption, the answer is clearly "yes."

By paying a little more attention to the brands you purchase, it's possible to make a significant difference in your overall calorie and fat consumption. Will making these types of changes cause you to lose 10 pounds in 48 hours or nine inches off your waist in thirty days? No, but it may cause you to lose 5 or 10 pounds in a year. And it will represent the loss of fat, not water. And that weight is more likely to stay lost, rather than return with friends.

Low fat versus fat free

Part of the retraining process, therefore, involves making good choices. There are presently thousands of food items that are available in regular, low fat and fat free versions.

We substitute reduced calorie if we think it's an acceptable substitute for the real thing. Otherwise, we adjust the amount we use. Eliminating any food group stokes up the deprivation/binge eating demons, so we haven't eliminated anything from our diet.

There are reports that, as a result of reduced fat choices, Americans have decreased the percentage of fat in our diets. But we are not losing weight. We are gaining weight. Fat free food is not calorie free food. The fat that is eliminated from the product is replaced with something else. Frequently, the fat is replaced with sugar. Just because a bag contains fat free chips, doesn't mean that you can eat the entire bag. If you eat excess calories in fat free food, the body will convert those excess calories into excess body fat. It's not simply what we eat, it's also how much we eat that controls our weight.

Extra-lean beef

One major change in our cooking is utilizing the low fat meat products that are becoming readily available. These products allow traditional home-cooked meals to be prepared without sacrificing flavor to achieve reduced calories and fat content. We use 96 percent extra-lean ground beef in all of our recipes.

If you decide after reading this book to make one single change in your life and forget everything else, this is the change to make.

Never, ever, use anything but 96 percent extra-lean ground beef.

Since ground beef is the basis of so many standard family recipes, the savings in calories achieved by using the leaner beef makes a tremendous difference in the daily calorie consumption.

Why does it make so much difference?

According to the Center for Science in the Public Interest, ground beef is the single most damaging food in the American diet. The average American consumes 27 pounds of ground beef a year, and it is the third largest source of saturated fat.

One problem with ground beef is the information printed on the label. Ground beef is generally labeled 85/15, 85 percent lean and 15 percent fat, or 90/10, 90 percent lean and 10 percent fat. The price of the ground beef naturally increases as the percent fat on the label decreases. How many of us are willing to spend the money on 96/4, extra-lean ground beef, when it's so much more expensive than 85/15 beef? After all, 85/15 is only 15 percent fat, right? That doesn't sound too bad.

Unfortunately, 85/15 ground beef is 15 percent fat *by weight* which is fairly useless information. The 85 percent lean, 15 percent fat information is usually in large, easily read type. If you look at the information on the nutrition label, however, you can determine that a four ounce serving of 85/15 ground beef contains 240 calories and that 150 of those calories come from fat. Let's do a little math.

150/240 = .625

Multiply by 100 to get the percentage.

.625 x 100 = 62.5%

The 85/15 ground beef may be 15 percent fat by weight, but it's *62.5 percent fat by calories.*

Table 10.2 shows the difference between percent fat by weight and percent fat by calories. It's an ugly surprise to discover that the 90/10 ground beef you naturally assumed was 10 percent fat by calories, is actually 47 percent fat by calories.

Ground Beef (SERVING SIZE 4 OUNCES)					
% LEAN BY WEIGHT	% FAT BY WEIGHT	CALORIES (TOTAL)	CALORIES (FROM FAT)	% LEAN BY CALORIES	% FAT BY CALORIES
80	20	290	200	31	69
85	15	240	150	38	62
90	10	190	90	53	47
96	04	130	25	81	19

Table 10.2

Why is ground beef responsible for such a high percent of the saturated fat in our diet? We're buying 85/15 or 90/10 ground beef and feeling virtuous, because we don't understand that the label on the ground beef isn't telling us what we think it is. Even the leanest grade of ground beef still gets 19 percent of its calories from fat.

If I'm on a typical, temporary diet, I could simply not eat beef while I'm trying to lose weight. But I'm not on a temporary diet, I'm making permanent changes in my eating habits. I'm not willing to give up beef forever. I am willing to pay for the leanest beef product available. I am willing to use ground beef in dishes that also contain vegetables and starches. These recipes allow the meat portion of the dish to be reduced to a calorically acceptable level without giving up the taste of beef that we want.

Extra-lean ground beef is more expensive, but other grades of beef simply contain too many calories and too much fat to be an option for me. It is possible to produce reasonable servings that contain acceptable calories and fat by using extra-lean ground beef.

Lean pork

We eat lots of pork; we just choose the leanest cuts available — the center-cut pork loin or the pork tenderloin. Since the calorie and fat content varies greatly between brands, it is necessary to purchase pork that carries a nutrition label. We try to buy pork with 100-120 calories and 3-4.5 grams of fat in a four-ounce portion. This pork compares favorably to chicken in calories with only a slightly higher fat content.

The most critical factor in preparing pork that tastes good is the cooking time. Concern about trichinosis and other worm organisms created a generation of cooks who overcooked pork with a vengeance. Pork was cooked to an internal temperature of 170° F and tasted like shoe leather.

It is now recognized that worm organisms are killed at an internal temperature of 137° F. Modern recommendations for cooking pork generally list 140° F as the safe temperature. Buy a meat thermometer and give pork a chance. You'll be pleasantly surprised.

The use of lean beef and lean pork enables us to significantly lower the calories in our recipes. The more recipes we altered, the easier it was to continue dieting successfully. These changes are not temporary changes. These are long-term changes to the recipes that compose our standard daily fare, our diet.

Milk

I used to drink two percent milk. I gradually weaned myself down to one percent, then 1/2 percent, and finally, skim. I drink milk, so I don't have osteoporosis when I'm an old lady, and because I love it. I trained myself to drink the lower calorie, lower fat version of this product. And I was willing to do so.

There are a variety of food items whose variation in calories is the result of using the various milk products. There is reduced calorie sour cream, cottage cheese and cream cheese, and fat free versions of the same products. I eat the reduced fat versions of these products. I'm not willing to use the fat free versions; I don't like the taste. But you should try them for yourself; you may disagree with me.

The milk label is similar to the ground beef label. Milk is another product whose label lists calorie by weight. Table 10.3 shows the calories in the various dairy products.

	CALORIES		CALORIES
SKIM MILK	80 / CUP	REDUCED FAT CREAM CHEESE	60 / OZ.
1% MILK	130 / CUP	REGULAR CREAM CHEESE	80 / OZ.
2% MILK	140 / CUP	LOW FAT SOUR CREAM	324 / CUP
3.5% MILK	160 / CUP	REGULAR SOUR CREAM	492 / CUP
HALF & HALF	317 / CUP	LOW FAT COTTAGE CHEESE	160 / CUP
MEDIUM CREAM	608 / CUP	REDUCED FAT COTTAGE CHEESE	200 / CUP
HEAVY CREAM	792 / CUP	REGULAR COTTAGE CHEESE	240 / CUP

Table 10.3

Cheese as a condiment

Perhaps no other single item in our diet was altered more than our consumption of cheese. Cheese is one of my favorite foods and I always purchased it in those handy eight-ounce packages. It never occurred to me that a casserole should be covered by anything less than an entire package.

Even if we use lower fat milk products, most of us manage to ignore the fact that most cheeses are "full-fat" dairy products. Cheese is a combination food, it contains both protein and fat. But, at 110 calories and nine grams of fat per ounce, the typical cheese is fairly comparable to any of the fats listed in Table 10.4. Cheese is a calorically dense food, and it's possible to add a tremendous number of calories and fat grams very quickly.

We use part-skim mozzarella and low fat ricotta. If a recipe calls for cheese, and mozzarella will give the right taste, it's a better calorie and fat choice than cheddar. Using sharp cheddar rather than mild or medium cheddar helps add the desired flavor without using as much cheese.

We didn't quit using cheese. We're just much more careful about the amount we use.

Fat

No discussion of changes in diet can be complete without discussing fat. The fat category encompasses oil, butter and mayonnaise. The table below lists calories and fat grams for common fats.

	CALORIES	FAT GRAMS	
Butter, one tablespoon	100	11	
Margarine, one tablespoon	100	11	
Vegetable Oil, one tablespoon	120	14	
Mayonnaise, one tablespoon	100	11	
Lard, one tablespoon	115	13	

Table 10.4

Cheese, fats, chocolate and nuts are all considered calorically dense foods, because the calorie to weight ratio is so high. It is, therefore, possible to consume massive number of calories without any satiation of hunger due the density of calories in these foods.

The presence of food labels helps make eating properly much easier. It provides a wealth of information about our food choices. It makes paying attention to the food we eat much easier, but deciding whether you're eating properly can still be a challenge. Sometimes it's necessary to understand exactly what standard has been set for a particular definition.

Food Claims

If a label advertises a food as being fat free, cholesterol free, low sodium, or high fiber, the food must meet well defined criteria. A food product labeled fat free, must have less than a half a gram of fat per serving; a product labeled calorie free, must have four or fewer calories per serving. If you consume a sufficient number of servings of products that are, per serving, considered to be both fat and calorie free, you may actually consume a significant amount of fat and calories. A cholesterol free product must have less than two milligrams per serving; carbohydrate, fiber, sugar or protein free products must have less than half a gram per serving.

If a food product claims to be low in some nutrient, or reduced, it must be in reference to a similar product. By definition, a reduced fat product must have 25 percent less fat than the comparable full fat product. So, a reduced fat cookie will have at least 25 percent less fat than the comparable regular cookie, but that doesn't necessarily qualify the cookie as low fat. A low fat item also must have less than three grams of fat per serving.

A low sodium product must have less than 140 milligrams of sodium per serving; a very low sodium product must have less than 35 milligrams of sodium per serving. This designation only applies to products that are not naturally low in sodium. Chicken broth is available as regular, low sodium, and very low sodium. Frozen or fresh corn is naturally low in sodium, so it is not labeled low or very low sodium. In order to make claims regarding low or reduced products, something must have been done to that product to make it that way.

Similarly, if a label states a product is fortified or enriched, it must have at least 10 percent more of the daily-recommended value of protein, vitamins, minerals, dietary fiber, or potassium, than some reference product. A good source must have 10-19 percent more, while a high source must have at least 20 percent more of the specific nutrient, than the reference product.

Things are less clear when the adjective used is light or lite. Technically, a light product indicates a product which normally derives more than 50 percent of its calories from fat has reduced its calories by at least 50 percent. Butter is a good example of this situation. Butter has 100 calories and 11 grams of fat per tablespoon, and it derives essentially all of its calories from fat. Light butter has 50 calories and six grams of fat in a tablespoon.

However, regular olive oil and light olive oil both have 120 calories and 14 grams of fat per tablespoon. Why? In this example, the light in the product description refers to the strength of the olive flavor in the oil. Light brown sugar refers to the color and molasses content of the brown sugar.

If you've never paid any attention to food labels, you'll be surprised how much easier they make it to keep track of your calories.

How did we lose so much weight? We were eating really well, so it was actually pretty painless. It just took time.

chapter 11

The Last Twelve Pounds

My previous weight of 247 pounds correlated with a BMI of 45.1 and the clinical definition of morbid obesity; my goal weight of 135 pounds correlated with a BMI of 24.7 and the clinical definition of normal weight. The journey from morbid obesity to normal weight represented 112 pounds.

How long did it take you to lose that much weight?

Well, it took a year and eight months to lose the first 100 pounds. And I've maintained that loss since February 2002.

What happened to the last twelve pounds?

Can I let you know later?

There was something magical sounding about losing one hundred pounds. But once I'd lost it, it became very difficult to get motivated to lose any more.

The loss of 100 pounds put me at a familiar weight. A weight I'd been numerous times in my life. I might have no idea which single instant I weighed 110 pounds, but there had been a lot of days when I had weighed 147. Was this a weight my body was comfortable with or a weight my mind was comfortable with? Or were other factors influencing my behavior?

What motivates us to diet? For women, concern about appearance receives the highest rank, followed by future health, then current health. For men, future health occupies the first position, followed by appearance and current health. And there are other external influences that can effect our proper weight decisions. One of these inanimate, but powerful objects is the scale.

Table 11.1 shows these motivators by percentage for both men and women.

	WOMEN	MEN
Appearance:	19%	18%
Future health:	21%	29%
Current health:	16%	16%

Table 11.1

In my previous reduced-calorie diet life, I had been obsessed by the scales. I weighed myself at least once a day. If I was dieting and having a bad day, I weighed myself multiple times. The worse I was, the more necessary the weigh-ins, as if weighing myself would provide tangible proof of the need for deprivation, and somehow stop the binging. If I was having a good day or several good days, I could be satisfied with a once-a-day weigh-in, but I expected instant response from the scales to prove that the sacrifices associated with dieting were being appropriately rewarded.

At lower weights, there is great power in a change in the 10's column of one's weight. When I was in high school, I weighed between 120 and 129 pounds. I never seemed to be able to get below 120, but whenever I got to 129 pounds, I managed to muster the will power to diet back down to 120. For me, the mental difference between 129 and 130 always seemed more significant than the physical difference between 120 and 129.

Now, once you pass 150 pounds, the change in the 10's column loses ground to the power of the 50-pound weight. Is there anything more horrible than watching while a finger gradually shifts the top weight further toward the 50 on the upper scale, while you pray for the arrow to fall? I'd moved past the 150-pound weight in my 30s, and I'd spent my 40s struggling to keep the 200-pound weight in play.

My 100-pound weight loss coincides with a weight that places me just below one of those critical weights. At 147 pounds, I have three pounds of cushion before the bottom weight on the scale will have to be moved from the 100-pound weight to the 150-pound weight. But I just can't get that excited about the last twelve pounds. I appear to have arrived at the weight I *can live with once I get there.*

Garment Tags

Clothing size can provide similar influence. But clothing size is more complicated than the weight shown on a set of scales. Scales are empirical devices that measure the effect of gravity on our earthbound bodies. The size displayed on a clothing tag *can* and *is* being manipulated.

In the 1970s, there was a voluntary effort by manufacturers to standardize women's sizes. The size 8 established by the PS 42-70 Standard fit dimensions of 33"-24"-35". The increasing size of today's population has made those standard fit dimensions completely outdated. A survey of 16 of today's women's apparel manufacturers indicated that the dimensions of today's size 8 are 36"-27"-37.5", an increase of 3 inches in the bust, 3 inches in the waist, and 2.5" in the hips over the 1970 standard. Yesterday's size 8 is today's size 4. Size 0s and 2s were created so that clothing with larger dimensions could still have acceptable numbers on the labels.

Who among us has not purchased a garment that was clearly larger than expected for the size on the tag? When I was wearing a size 14, I tried on a blouse. It was unexpectedly large. I tried the size 12. I tried the size 10. Finally, the size eight fit. I bought the blouse.

A tape measure would surely have demonstrated that the dimensions of that blouse were identical to another manufacturer's size 14, but I couldn't help being seduced by the size 8 on the label. Even though I knew the size on the tag wasn't accurate, I still bought the blouse. I stood in the store and discussed with Diane how incorrect the tag was, but I still bought the blouse.

Even now, my weight decisions are influenced by external factors. Just under the 150-pound weight on the scales and wearing jeans with size six tags, it's difficult to care that the BMI chart insists I'm still overweight. After losing 100 pounds, it's difficult to care enough about the last 12 pounds to lose them.

Why did I quit losing weight? I've reached a place that my mind thinks is acceptable, and I've reached a place where my body is in caloric equilibrium. I'm eating the same number of calories that my body is expending in basic metabolic processes and physical activity.

I'm obviously eating a few more calories than my designated 1,600, because I've stabilized at slightly higher weight than my original goal weight of 135 pounds. But my weight has stabilized. I've quit losing weight, but I haven't started regaining the weight that I had lost. In the process of losing one hundred pounds I have made permanent changes in my eating habits.

Have I learned to eat properly? I've certainly learned to eat tremendously better than when I started. And I've arrived at an interesting place. Instead of being morbidly obese, I am now one of those annoying women who complain about needing to lose twelve pounds.

Why is it so hard to lose the last 10 or 12 pounds?

How much am I eating if my weight has stabilized at 147 pounds?

147 pounds x 12 calories/pound = 1,764 calories

What would I be eating to weigh 135 pounds?

135 pounds x 12 calories/pound = 1,620 calories

The difference between the two weights?

1764 calories – 1620 calories = 144 calories

The caloric difference between weighing 147 pounds and weighing 135 pounds is a measly 144 calories per day.

Why is no one in America happy with their weight? Why does everyone have at least ten or twenty pounds they want to lose?

Because there's not very much caloric difference between ten pound intervals of weight.

How much food is 144 calories?

It's approximately:
• 35 peanuts
• 1 tablespoon of butter and 1 1/2 tablespoons of sour cream
• 17 jellybeans
• 1 1/2 tablespoons of mayonnaise
• 34 candy-coated chocolate candies
• 8 reduced-fat wheat crackers and 3/4 ounce of cheese
• 7 sourdough hard pretzels

It's really easy to eat an extra 144 calories a day. Or an extra 288 calories a day.

If I manage to rustle up enough resolve to reduce my caloric intake by that 144 calories, how long will it take me to reach 135 pounds?

3,500 calories/pound /144 calories/day = 24 days/pound
24 days/pound x 12 pounds = 288 days

Assuming 30 days per month, it'll take me almost 10 months to lose 12 pounds.

Will I lose the next twelve pounds? Can I get back to you on that? The dream weight is 135 pounds. It represents a 45 percent decrease in body weight. I'm hanging in there at 100 pounds lost, a decrease of 40 percent. Should I feel bad? I don't think so. Especially since I'm healthy.

As a 47 year-old, morbidly obese woman, I was extraordinarily lucky. Through nothing but genetic good luck, I had none of the health risks associated with being overweight and obese. I am fortunate enough to have parents who are both 82 years old and in fairly good health. Despite fighting his own battles with weight, my father has always had low blood pressure, and I obviously inherited his genes. I knew, however, that the older I became, the more likely I was to develop health problems.

What should we be doing to improve our health besides improve our diets? We need to be getting some exercise. Get off the couch, turn off the TV, and get your body moving.

My body? It may not be a normal weight, but it's moving.

chapter 12

The Evil Empire of Exercise

In June 2000, we were primarily interested in losing weight. Ultimately, however, our goals shifted. We became less interested in the final number on the scales and became more interested in our overall health. Despite disagreement on the exact relationship between diet and exercise, there's little disagreement among health professionals that moderate physical activity is an important component of a healthy lifestyle. This is true whether or not you're trying to lose weight. If you are trying to lose weight, it is even more important to exercise.

In order to maximize the loss of fat and protect muscle mass, you must exercise while dieting. If you diet without exercising, the ratio of fat to muscle loss may be as low as 80 percent fat, 20 percent muscle. If you exercise, the ratio of fat to muscle loss can be as high as 95 percent fat, five percent muscle. If you're serious not only about losing weight, but also about improving your health, dieting without exercise isn't an option.

Why should you care about your muscle mass? Because the more body weight derived from muscle, the more calories you get to consume. That's right. More calories. Our muscle cells are the most metabolically active tissue in the body; our lean muscle mass burns calories. The better your body's ratio of lean muscle to fat, the more calories your body burns, whether you're walking on a treadmill or sitting on a sofa. If you reduce your lean muscle mass, you decrease your body's ability to metabolize calories.

What about fat? Fat is essentially inert. Fat spends its days doing nothing.

Fat cells are couch potatoes at the molecular level!

Remember the 12 calories per pound formula? The formula was based on an inactive person. If you exercise while you're losing weight, you not only lose weight more quickly, you also increase your muscle mass. Once you get to your goal weight, you'll be able to eat more while maintaining your weight. You'll be burning calories while exercising, and your body will have more metabolically active muscle tissue.

If you are female, you have a naturally higher percentage of body fat and less muscle mass. Since women are normally shorter and smaller-framed, it also takes fewer calories to maintain a normal weight. Making exercise part of your daily life allows you to eat a few more calories and still stay within the normal weight range.

Life used to provide plenty of exercise, but modern life provides very little. Food is more readily available, and most of us no longer lead lives that require the level of caloric intake that we consume. A hundred years ago, we were a society of farmers and laborers whose day-to-day survival depended on hard physical labor. Today, we are a nation of sedentary office workers who use telephones, computers and automobiles to conduct our business. Women no longer scrub clothes down by the riverside and hang them outside to dry. Chicken dinner doesn't start with a chicken pecking seeds in the backyard, but with chicken fried at the fast food restaurant.

If our jobs no longer require physical labor, exercise must be incorporated into our leisure-time schedules. However, recent government statistics indicate that 40 percent of adults engage in no leisure-time physical activity. None. Nada. Zip. Additionally, only fifteen percent of adults presently meet the government recommendations of regular moderate physical activity for at least 30 minutes per day.

Why do the government recommendations for health include recommendations for physical activity?

Regular physical activity is beneficial to maintaining a normal weight, but its benefits extend far beyond weight control. Regular exercise improves our blood lipid profile. It lowers our blood cholesterol, removes cholesterol deposits from the walls of blood vessels, and reduces our risk from heart attack and stroke. Regular exercise improves our endurance by improving the condition of our muscles, including our heart and lungs. Exercise helps us stay active as we age, by maintaining joint flexibility and by preserving bone mass which prevents osteoporosis.

I'd been a lifetime member of the Coach Potato Hall of Fame, and I went kicking and screaming into a pair of gym shoes. I could spell exercise, but I didn't like to get that close to it. And as far as I was concerned, sweat was what formed on the outside of a wine glass on a warm day.

For the first eight weeks, all we did was diet. For those 56 days, the most important thing was staying on the diet. After eight weeks we started exercising. We started by walking around the neighborhood. The first few weeks were tremendously pitiful. I whined while I walked, and my thigh muscles twitched in horrified protest at the scorching one-mile per hour pace. We gradually, very gradually, increased the pace. We walked four to five times a week. At the end of the first year, we were walking three miles in an hour, and we wanted to vary our routine, so we joined an athletic club.

Yesterday, I spent thirty-five minutes on a cross-trainer and twenty-five minutes on an elliptical trainer. I'm living proof that it's possible to exercise without loving it. You don't even have to like it very much. I don't. You do need to feel guilty, if you don't do it. It needs to be like brushing your teeth, washing the makeup off your face at night, and wearing clean underwear every morning. It needs to be on the list of things you do. Period.

Unfortunately, the heavier we are, the more difficult exercise may be. The less we exercise, the less muscle we maintain, and a cycle of weight gain accompanied by less and less activity can develop. *If you have significant health problems associated with being overweight, your primary care physician should make recommendations before you begin any exercise regimen.*

The most important thing is to do something. Do as much you can, but be sensible. Don't overdo. It's far more important to do a little each day, day after day, than to do too much on any one day. You'll get hurt and quit. The remarkable thing is that if you continue to do a little each day, then a little more each day, you suddenly discover you can do more than you ever thought possible.

Exercising needs to be as much a habit as eating a proper diet. Exercise needs to be part of a permanent change in your lifestyle. The rewards can be amazing. It is truly remarkable that my body could forgive the years of abuse to which it had been subjected. I'd been morbidly obese for a decade, but my body didn't hold it against me.

Brett and I went to Hilton Head Island, and we rode a tandem bicycle all over the island. Diane and I went to New York City and walked for blocks. We walked for hours, when we previously couldn't have walked for more than a few minutes.

Am I thin? No. But I'm in the best physical shape of my life.

Fit vs. Fat

There are numerous medical professionals who argue against the focus on weight. They insist that fitness, not fatness, is the crucial element in determining health. And even if being overweight is identified as a health risk for certain diseases, is it significant in an individual with no risk factors?

The situation is complicated because definitive correlations between weight and health are impossible to empirically establish. While it is generally agreed that morbid obesity is unhealthy, it is not clear at what point excess weight stops being a health risk and becomes a health problem.

There are studies that indicate overweight individuals who exercise may be healthier than individuals of proper weights who do not exercise. But most people who are overweight do not exercise. Although it is theoretically possible for people to be fit and fat, it is not the norm.

At 147 pounds, my BMI does not classify me for the normal weight category, but I am extremely fit. When I weighed 247 pounds, I was not fit. And there was no way I was going to become fit at that weight. In order to be able to do the physical activities that would help me become fit, I first had to lose weight.

So, you're learning new proper eating habits. You're losing weight. You're exercising. Do you feel good about yourself? You should.

If you can only be happy when you get thin thighs, you may be doomed to disappointment. There are certain unpleasant truths that need to be addressed when discussing exercise and weight loss. Losing weight does not change the basic shape of our bodies, it just makes the basic shape smaller. A great deal of our body habitus is genetically ordained.

There have been innumerable people who have become rich selling potions, creams, and a wide variety of machines that promise to remove fat from a specific area of the body. But fat is systemic. This means that the charming bulges on the outside of your thighs, my thighs, and everyone else's thighs, is fat that just happens to be stored on the outside of the thighs. It is visiting your thighs, but it is not thigh fat. It is body fat. It is fat that is being stored by the body to provide energy when the next great famine or diet begins. The only way to lose fat from your thighs is to lose fat from your entire body. And even after you lose a great deal of weight, you may still have thigh bulges.

In order to have washboard abs or a buff butt or not have old lady, batwing arms, first you have to lose the excess body fat. After you've lost the excess body fat, you have to tone specific muscle groups to produce the sculptured musculature that all endorsers of diet products seem to have magically obtained without diet or exercise.

If Hollywood is to provide our standard for physical beauty, we need to be objective in our analysis of that standard. Based on the body mass index charts, most of the female Hollywood population is underweight. In addition to non-standard heights and weights, the number of Hollywood physiques who owe a great deal to multi-hour per day workouts is considerable. For each genetically blessed individual, there is another rigidly disciplined personality who watches every calorie and spends hours with a personal trainer.

Most women who are underweight are not particularly well endowed. I would have to weight less than 101 pounds to be underweight; at that weight, my chest would probably be concave. Based on this personal observation, the underweight Hollywood population is either genetically or surgically blessed. And, in addition to breast implants, surgeons can change noses, chins, cheekbones and a myriad of other flaws. How much of what we compare ourselves to is a surgical illusion assisted by makeup, hair extensions and designer clothing?

So, even though I've lost more than a hundred pounds, I still have to periodically remind myself that I'm not ever going to look like Catherine Zeta-Jones. And that I'm not ever going to have thin thighs. But losing weight and exercising has given me things far more valuable. It's given me the ability to climb flights of stairs without gasping for breath. It's given me the energy to walk beside my husband without needing him to slow down. It's given me hope for a longer, healthier life.

It's even given me thinner thighs.

chapter 13

Sharing a Miracle –
The Temple Reconstruction Project

L osing 100 pounds was the answer to more than one desperate prayer for help. But it was, quite frankly, an unexpected answer. Losing twenty pounds would have been a satisfactory answer. Losing 50 pounds would have been a great answer. Losing 100 pounds? That was a miracle.

We had been dieting for a year by the summer of 2001. We were incorporating the theories of *Eucalorics* into our lives. We were dieting and losing weight; we had started working on this book. Brett was reading, I was writing and Diane was cooking.

Our lives changed when a close friend, David Bondurant, had a stroke. Medically, the symptoms were all resolved, so it was classified as a TIA, a transient ischemic attack. But David's personal physician issued another in a long line of warnings. David had multiple health problems: high cholesterol, high blood pressure, and type 2 diabetes that were all aggravated by excess weight. The TIA was a warning. If David did not change his eating habits and lifestyle, he was clearly at risk for a more serious stroke that might either disable him or kill him. David's wife, whose name is also Jackie, left the doctor's office and began to pray for help.

When Brett told Diane and I about David's TIA, we offered to begin cooking for David and Jackie. Our ideas and recipes were working well for us, perhaps they would also work for David. Initially, David and Jackie were concerned that cooking for them would be too much work. After some discussion, we agreed that we would try it. If it became too much trouble, we would tell them. We began to cook for David and Jackie in July 2001, and they gradually began to lose weight.

Eucalorics

Jackie didn't tell us until much later about her prayers. We, who had received an answer to our own prayers, had become the answer to someone else's prayers. We were given a chance to share our miracle.

We sing in our church choir, and choir members who had been watching our family lose weight were now watching David and Jackie lose weight as well. People started to ask, "Are you going to start cooking for anybody else?" In January 2002, our church gave us permission to use their commercial kitchen. We recruited a small group and started the Temple Reconstruction Project.

Do you not know that your body is a temple of the Holy Spirit, who is in you, whom you have received from God? You are not your own.

1 Corinthians 6:19

Our little group had chef surprise every night, while we experimented with techniques and recipes. We planned to cook for twelve weeks. Twelve weeks was followed by another twelve weeks. Then another.

Three weeks into the project, the church cook quit, and we suddenly inherited dinner for 120 people every Wednesday night, in addition to our dieters. We cooked for special dinners and Holy Week lunches and Vacation Bible School. In the fall of 2003, the Wednesday Night Dinners are averaging 170 people.

We cooked for dieters in the basement of the First United Methodist Church for a year and a half. Our dieters came to the basement of the church and picked up dinner four nights a week. Dinner that was weighed and measured and labeled. The recipes in this book are the result of feeding real people, real food, night after night. They are the result of having real people say, *too spicy, too dry, too much, too little.* They were developed in the "test kitchen" of our church.

Our youngest patron was two. While her parents were trying to learn new eating habits, Katie started life with good eating habits. Katie eats carrots, broccoli and asparagus. She eats chicken, meatloaf and pork roast. She got 1/2 of an adult portion, and she learned to eat food the average two-year-old didn't, because this was the food she was given. Katie thought fast food came from the basement at the First United Methodist Church.

How did we lose so much weight and keep it off? We ate well. Monday through Friday, we cooked two different meals. And every night I had trouble deciding which of the two meals I wanted for dinner. Every night I sat down and ate a meal that tasted good. Every night I ate a meal that kept my head and my body happy. We continue to eat meals that keep us content.

We know you're busy. We know you're eating lots of meals out. We include a list of eating out options in the back of this book, but we're hoping you'll try some of these recipes. You may be pleasantly surprised to find recipes for real food in a diet book.

The recipes in most diet books are constrained by either food group or calorie count. When those constraints are removed, and careful food choice and preparation are included, it's possible to have recipes for real food. If you've been trying to subsist on diet meal rations, it means more food. Lots more food.

When we talked to people about losing weight, they were fascinated by the idea of eating to support a goal weight. It made so much sense to lose weight while learning how to maintain your weight loss. And people simply couldn't believe the quantity and quality of the food they can eat and still lose weight.

We usually try to lose weight by starving ourselves. It doesn't work. Eating the correct number of calories in the proper portions creates new eating habits that can be followed forever. *Eucalorics* represents a means to achieve and maintain a normal weight.

chapter 14

Consider the Alternatives

Yₒu are almost finished with the first portion of the book. Ask yourself if the ideas sound intriguing. Are you ready to jump right in on *Day One*? Ready to start looking at meal plans and recipes? Or are you overwhelmed?

Are you thinking to yourself, how nice for them that they lost so much weight, but they cook and exercise. That's not happening in my life. I was hoping for a weight loss miracle.

You purchased this book, so you're obviously not happy with your weight. How unhappy are you? What else could you try?

You could decide you don't care about being overweight.

The anti-diet movement presents an alternate response to the widespread failure of traditional weight loss. Concerned with the psychological frustrations associated with continued failure, these groups focus on changing public attitudes towards the overweight population.

It is certainly true that in a country that strives to eliminate all forms of intolerance, discrimination against fat people is alive and well. A now famous article in the February 1994 issue of *Esquire* indicated that women between the ages of 18 and 25 would rather be run over by a truck than be extremely fat. Two-thirds would choose to be mean or stupid, rather than to be fat.

The National Association to Advance Fat Acceptance (NAAFA) is one organization that lobbies against such attitudes. In an ideal world, no one would suffer from any form of discrimination, but the ethical stance that requires protection for the legal and moral rights of overweight individuals does not address the health issues associated with being overweight.

We live in a society that expects a legal solution to exist for every problem, but it won't help me long-term to pass a law which makes it illegal to discriminate based on my weight, if I die of a heart attack when I'm 50. It's not possible to pass a law that mandates protection from the medical consequences of obesity. The morbidly obese who have the greatest need of protection from discrimination are the individuals most likely to have serious health consequences as a result of their excess weight.

You could decide to focus on maintaining your present weight.

The changes in the Dietary Guidelines for Americans are, quite frankly, headed in that direction. The lack of success from both traditional and non-traditional diets has been so far reaching that there is starting to be real concern that losing weight is impossible, or at least unlikely. As categorized below, the changing expectations regarding weight expressed by the dietary guidelines.

- Maintain ideal weight
- Maintain desirable weight
- Maintain healthy weight
- Balance the food you eat with physical activity; maintain or improve your weight
- Aim for a healthy weight — be physically active every day

The problem with deciding that maintaining weight is sufficient is that even maintenance can be difficult without making some changes. I had long held a personal theory (completely unencumbered by facts) that there was a static amount of weight in the world. If one person was losing weight, there was someone else gaining it. I was obviously personally responsible for some spectacular losses by some unknown person or persons. Occasionally, when I was on a losing streak, I was sure I was being balanced out by some poor out-of-control soul temporarily engaged in unbridled feasting.

I have been forced to question the validity of that theory based on two events. First, the ugly statistics which indicate that NO ONE in America is losing weight, and next, the complete failure of my second personal theory.

That was the theory that clung to the hope there was some upper limit at which my own personal weight gain would level off. I had accepted that it was going to be a spectacularly, overwhelmingly, enormously HUGE weight. But, when I reached it, I could at least quit worrying about gaining more weight and only deal with being really, really (really) fat.

Sad to report, however, such a weight did not appear to exist. My own weight had gradually increased until my final mental barrier involved the very real possibility that I would exceed 250 pounds. Whenever my weight approached 250 pounds, I would engage in one more round of dieting. I had spent my 30s struggling between 150 pounds and 200 pounds. During my 40s, the battle had moved to the 200 and 250 pounds level, and the last few years, I had remained at the upper end of the range. At that rate, I could look forward to 500 pounds at age 80. Even at that weight, I still wouldn't be in the running for the Guinness Book of World Records for fatness, but, quite frankly, that had never been one of my life's goals.

Would making small changes in my diet have allowed me to lose some weight or at least maintain my weight? Probably, but I wasn't happy with the idea of maintaining my weight, I wanted to be thin.

At this point, I no longer feel the need to be thin. I've reached a weight that still is technically overweight for my height, but it's a weight I can live with. It's a weight I can maintain.

If you think you can make small changes, but not make drastic changes, then make small changes. Making small changes will probably not only help you maintain your present weight, but also will probably help you lose some weight.

Start with the following list of small changes. Make as many of the following changes as possible.

Do not tell yourself or anyone else you are on a new diet.
You're not on a diet. You're making some small changes in your daily fare.

1. Don't plan to start a diet. Eat what you've been eating, but don't plan to start a diet on Monday. Since you're not planning to diet, you won't need to spend the weekend doing "Last Supper" eating. You won't need to eat a gallon of ice cream or boxes of cookies in preparation for the famine scheduled to arrive at 8 a.m. Monday morning.

2. Eat breakfast every day. Pick things you like from the breakfast list and eat breakfast every day.

3. Eat at least one piece of fruit every day. Not fruit juice. Fruit. If you consistently eat one piece of fruit, start trying to eat two. Aim for variety.

4. Eat at least two servings of vegetables every day. If you are consistently eating two servings, start trying to eat three. Aim for variety.

5. Consume the skim and low-fat versions of dairy products. Drink skim milk. Why? Fewer calories. Less fat.

6. When using ground beef, use only 96 percent extra lean ground beef. Why? Fewer calories. Less fat.

7. If you drink real soda, calculate how much you drink each day. Reduce it by half. Consider changing to diet soda.

8. Eat at fast food chains that offer salads. Before you eat anything else, eat a salad with either low-fat dressing or full-fat dressing on the side.

9. When you eat fast food — if you normally super-size your meal, stop. If you don't normally super-size, but you do order a combination meal, don't order the combination meal. Instead, order the sandwich you normally eat, but order a small fry.

10. Make as many small food changes as you can, and start walking a little bit every day.

Will this list of "To Do's" make your diet perfect? No. But the chances are pretty good that it will improve it.

Still seem like too much? Pick one thing on the list. Do it for a week. Add one more. Do them both for a week. Keep going until you're doing all ten. You've probably noticed that I'm in favor of starting with whatever seems possible. It's better to make some improvement than no improvement.

Or, you could decide to have surgery.

If you're morbidly obese, bariatric surgery is one solution to your weight problems. It's not a solution either Diane or I ever considered. Both of us would have been considered "good" candidates for this type of surgery. But I wasn't even willing to consider a food group restricting diet, so giving up food forever didn't seem to be a viable option. And, since I'm married to a surgeon, I was more aware than the average person of the risks associated with this type of procedure.

What do you get to eat after weight loss surgery? Take a look at the post-surgical diet of a gastric bypass patient.

Days 1-3   **Intravenous liquids**

Days 3-10   **Clear Liquids**
• Low sodium broth
• Sugar-free flavored gelatin
• Lemonade
• Fruit juice, except orange, pineapple or tomato
• Decaffeinated coffee or tea

Days 10-17   **Full Liquids**
Everything on clear liquid diet, plus
• Cooked cereals
• Strained soups
• Skim milk
• Plain yogurt
• Orange, pineapple and tomato juice
• Sugar-free pudding

Days 17-25   **Pureed Food**
Everything on the clear and full liquid diet, plus
• Pureed fruits and vegetables
• Pureed cooked meats
• Poached or soft cooked eggs

Once you graduate to the regular diet, you can look forward to days whose food consumption looks like this:

8:00 a.m.
        1 ounce lean meat or 1 egg
        1/2 bread serving
        1 teaspoon diet margarine

9:15 a.m.
> 4 ounces juice, consumed over 40-60 minutes

11:00 a.m.
> 1 ounce skim milk
> 1/2 bread serving or 1 ounce cereal

12:15 p.m.
> 4 ounces skim milk, consumed over 40-60 minutes

2:00 p.m.
> 1/2 bread or starch serving
> 2 ounces lean meat or protein
> 1 ounce diet margarine

3:15 p.m.
> 4 ounces vegetable or vegetable juice

5:00 p.m.
> 1/2 bread or starch serving
> 1 ounce lean meat or protein
> 1 ounce vegetable
> 1 teaspoon diet margarine

6:15 p.m.
> 4 ounces skim milk, consumed over 40-60 minutes

8:00 p.m.
> 4 ounces fruit

9:30 p.m.
> 1/2 bread serving
> 1 ounce skim milk

If you are extremely heavy and learn to eat properly, you will lose weight by making significant and permanent changes in your eating habits.

If you are extremely heavy and have bariatric surgery, you will lose weight by making significant and permanent changes in your eating habits.

Yesterday, I ate 1,600 calories. I had a chocolate chip muffin for breakfast, a Greek salad with hummus for lunch and chicken cacciatore for dinner. Plus snacks.

Take a look at the menus in Part Two. Take another look at a day in the life of a bariatric surgery patient.

Am I a perfect eater? No. Do I have days when I eat more than my daily-allotted calories? Yes. But, I spend time on an elliptical trainer, and I have more days when I eat properly than days when I eat improperly. And, I have the option of going to New York and eating fabulous food for three days, without being physically ill. And, I can choose to have cheesecake for dinner tonight by spending an hour on a cross-trainer in the morning. I haven't given up eating normally forever in order to be thin.

Our goal in writing this book is to provide tools and encouragement that will help you live in today's fat food world. This world is not perfect, but it's the only world we have. Try to make changes that will allow you to live a longer, happier and healthier life in this imperfect world.

chapter 15

The Pyramid Plan

I n Chapter Three, we computed the number of calories that would sustain your goal weight. For convenience, we repeat that computation here.

Goal Weight in pounds = _____.

Female:

_____ x 12 calories/pounds/day = _____ calories/day
Weight in pounds

Male:

_____ x 14 calories/pounds/day = _____ calories/day
Weight in pounds

This formula provides your daily caloric allotment — the number of calories that you need to consume each day in order to achieve and maintain your goal weight.

Table 15.1 lists daily caloric intake.

My goal weight is 135 pounds, and my daily caloric allotment is 1,620 calories. How do I consume my calories?

Calories have been calculated as follows:

DAILY CALORIC INTAKE - WOMEN				
LBS CALORIES	LBS CALORIES	LBS CALORIES	LBS CALORIES	LBS CALORIES
100 1200	125 1500	150 1800	175 2100	200 2400
105 1260	130 1560	155 1860	180 2160	205 2460
110 1320	135 1620	160 1920	185 2220	210 2520
115 1380	140 1680	165 1980	190 2280	215 2580
120 1440	145 1740	170 2040	195 2340	220 2640
DAILY CALORIC INTAKE - MEN				
LBS CALORIES	LBS CALORIES	LBS CALORIES	LBS CALORIES	LBS CALORIES
150 2100	175 2450	200 2800	225 3150	250 3550
155 2170	180 2520	205 2870	230 3270	255 3620
160 2240	185 2590	210 2940	235 3340	260 3690
165 2310	190 2660	215 3010	240 3410	265 3760
170 2380	195 2730	220 3080	245 3480	270 3830

Table 15.1

Table 15.2 shows daily caloric allotment by 100-calorie increments from 1,200 to 3,600. I use 1,600 calories a day as my daily caloric intake goal, and my caloric allotment is highlighted on Table 15.2.

Breakfast   10-20 percent total calories.
Lunch   25-30 percent total calories
Dinner   30-35 percent total calories
Snacks   15-30 percent total calories

CALORIES	BREAKFAST	LUNCH	DINNER	SNACKS
1200	120 - 240	300 - 360	360 - 420	180 - 360
1300	130 - 260	325 - 390	390 - 455	195 - 390
1400	140 - 280	350 - 420	420 - 490	210 - 420
1500	150 - 300	375 - 450	450 - 525	225 - 450
1600	160 - 320	400 - 480	480 - 560	240 - 480
1700	170 - 340	425 - 510	510 - 595	255 - 510
1800	180 - 360	450 - 540	540 - 630	270 - 540
1900	190 - 380	475 - 570	570 - 665	285 - 570
2000	200 - 400	500 - 600	600 - 700	300 - 600
2100	210 - 420	525 - 630	630 - 735	315 - 630
2200	220 - 440	550 - 660	660 - 770	330 - 660
2300	230 - 460	575 - 690	690 - 805	345 - 690
2400	240 - 480	600 - 720	720 - 840	360 - 720
2500	250 - 500	625 - 750	750 - 875	375 - 750
2600	260 - 520	650 - 780	780 - 910	390 - 780
2700	270 - 540	675 - 810	810 - 945	405 - 810
2800	280 - 560	700 - 840	840 - 980	420 - 840
2900	290 - 580	725 - 870	870 - 1015	435 - 870
3000	300 - 600	750 - 900	900 - 1050	450 - 900
3100	310 - 620	775 - 930	930 - 1085	465 - 930
3200	320 - 640	800 - 960	960 - 1120	480 - 960
3300	330 - 660	825 - 990	990 - 1155	495 - 990
3400	340 - 680	850 - 1020	1020 - 1190	510 - 1020
3500	350 - 700	875 - 1050	1050 - 1225	525 - 1050
3600	360 - 720	900 - 1080	1080 - 1260	540 - 1080
3700	370 - 740	925 - 1110	1110 - 1295	555 - 1110
3800	380 - 760	950 - 1140	1140 - 1330	570 - 1140

Table 15.2

Breakfast

Breakfast has been assigned 10-20 percent of my daily caloric allotment. I have a range of 160-320 calories for breakfast.

There's a good chance that you just thought to yourself, *Great, I'll have lots of calories for later in the day, since I never eat breakfast.*

How do I know that? In my former life, breakfast was the easiest meal to skip. I'm not a morning person, so I was always in a hurry. Besides, if I skipped breakfast I could bank those calories for later, right?

Ninety percent of the overweight population routinely skips one to two meals a day, and breakfast is the meal most commonly skipped, but skipping breakfast is associated with overweight, rather than normal weight.

Statistics demonstrate that the people who eat breakfast generally weigh less than those of us who don't eat breakfast.

Why is skipping a meal counterproductive? First, when we do begin eating, we overeat, more than compensating for those saved calories. Second, we sabotage our natural metabolic response to eating. When we eat, the body utilizes energy to digest, absorb and metabolize the nutrients contained in the food. Dietary-induced thermogenesis, increased metabolic rate as a result of eating, reaches a maximum approximately one hour after a meal. Skipping meals tends to decrease our metabolic rate.

The greatest decrease in metabolic rate occurs during sleep. Breakfast literally means to "break a fast," and eating following the period of fasting associated with sleep, provides a critical stimulus to the metabolism. The traditional wisdom that breakfast is the most important meal of the day is, therefore, backed up by present day scientific knowledge.

The proverbial excuse for not eating breakfast is lack of time. Make time. There are many quick and easy, take and go options, and we provide some in the meals and menus section of the book. If you're serious about learning to eat properly, the first absolute is breakfast. If you've never eaten breakfast, breakfast can be a small meal. But you need to learn to eat something. Breakfast is mandatory.

My stomach was initially quite surprised to get something besides Diet Dr Pepper® for breakfast. Now it expects it.

Lunch

Lunch receives 25-30 percent of my daily calorie allotment, or 400-480 calories. Since most of us aren't home to eat lunch, it can be a challenge to stay within this calorie window. If you pack a lunch, you're assured control over calories, but there is plenty of nutritional information available for eating out. Most fast food establishments have information posted in the restaurant or on their Web site.

Diane and I cook dinner five nights a week, but we frequently eat out at lunch. It is possible to achieve and maintain a normal weight while eating out, but you have to become an educated consumer. You have to know how many calories are in the food you are eating. And you have to be able to eat out without feeling deprived, or you'll create a situation that encourages overeating or binging because you're feeling sorry for yourself.

Dinner

For most of us, dinner is the main meal of the day. It receives 30-35 percent of the daily caloric allotment, so I have 480-560 calories for dinner. Whether I eat out or prepare a meal at home, dinner needs to be a meal, not an entrée. Dinner should consist of a protein, a starch and a vegetable.

If you look at our menus, you'll notice that we plan meals. Why? We need to eat meals that leave our heads and our bodies happy with the amount of food we've just consumed.

Snacks/Adjustments

This category receives a significant amount of calories, and the greatest range of calories, 15-30 percent. I've got 240-480 calories for either snacking or making adjustments to my other meals. This range of calories recognizes that in the world of eating, one size does not fit all. We have different lifestyles, different needs. We need to be able to have some flexibility in our meal and snack selection. These calories provide that flexibility.

If life were easy, we would make consistent food choices, so our bodies could be trained to eat approximately the same amount of food at the same time. But life is not easy, and it's hard to be consistent. We recommend trying to keep at least the pattern of your day consistent. Try to eat a core number of calories at each meal or snack. Beyond the core calories, adjust additional calories to suit your particular lifestyle and pattern of eating. You know what time of day, and in what situations, you have problems with food.

Do you want more calories at breakfast? Pick the high end of the range (20 percent of your calories), and then add an additional 10 percent from your snack allotment to allow a larger breakfast. Do you frequently eat out at lunch? Maybe you need extra calories there. Would it make sense for your dinner calories and lunch calories to be switched? Do you need to have an evening snack? Plan your day accordingly. Take a look at your own life and use the snack and adjustment calories to make the daily calorie allotment work for you. If you know you're going out for a special dinner, make minor adjustments in your daily schedule in order to compensate. Don't skip a meal or snack that you normally eat.

I find it is easiest to be mentally and physically happy eating 1,600 calories a day, if I eat consistently and frequently. I don't eat nearly as much at each meal, so I eat more often. A normal day in my life is presently divided as follows.

Breakfast	200-300 calories
Mid-morning snack	100 calories
Lunch	400-450 calories
Mid-afternoon snack	200-300 calories
Dinner	450-550 calories
Evening snack	100-200 calories

*How can I know what a **proper portion** is?*

The Food Pyramid, indicates that 6-11 servings of carbohydrates should be consumed, but the definitions of serving sizes and additional information about choosing the appropriate number from the given range are not located on The Pyramid. You have to look further. The Pyramid was not designed as a stand-alone source, but as one part of a package of information. The information on servings sizes for the various food groups is summarized in below.

Bread, Cereal, Rice and Pasta
1 slice bread
1 ounce of ready-to-eat cereal
1/2 cup cooked rice
1/2 cup cooked pasta

Vegetable
1 cup of raw leafy vegetables
1/2 cup other vegetables, cooked or chopped raw
3/4 cup of vegetable juice

Fruit
1 medium apple, banana, or orange
1/2 cup of chopped, cooked, or canned fruit
3/4 cup of fruit juice

Milk, Yogurt and Cheese
1 cup of milk or yogurt
1 1/2 ounces of natural cheese
2 ounces of processed cheese

Meat, Poultry, Fish, Dry Beans, Eggs and Nuts
2-3 ounces lean meat, poultry, or fish
1/2 cup of cooked dry beans = 1 ounce lean meat
1 egg = 1 ounce lean meat
2 tablespoons peanut butter = 1 ounce lean meat
1/3 cup nuts = 1 ounce of lean meat

Fats
1 teaspoon oil, butter, or margarine = a serving

Once you become familiar with servings sizes, you need to be aware of how many servings of each food group are appropriate for your individual caloric intake. There's a balancing act between getting appropriate nutrition and staying within the calories allotted to maintain your desired weight. The fewer the calories it takes to sustain your desired weight, the more difficult the balancing act becomes.

Table 15.3 lists the suggested servings of each food group for a diet of 1,600 calories, 2,200 calories, and 2,800 calories.

FOOD GROUP	1600 CALORIES	2200 CALORIES	2800 CALORIES
GRAINS	6	9	11
VEGETABLE	3	4	5
FRUIT	2	3	4
MILK	2 OR 3	2 OR 3	2 OR 3
MEAT	5 oz. total	6 oz. total	7 oz. total

Table 15.3

Do I have to count calories?

We do. We keep a food journal, and we count calories. When we started both the journal and the calorie count were kept on paper. Now, we keep a running tally in our heads. At any given moment, I know how many calories I've eaten; how many calories I have left. It's become a habit.

If you follow our menus and use our recipes, a great deal of the calorie counting has already been done for you. We've given you 28 days of meals. Twenty-eight breakfasts. Twenty-eight lunches. Twenty-eight dinners. All with calorie information.

Most people simply don't bother with that much variety in their lives. They pick two or three of the breakfasts, two or three of the lunches, and, introduce some variety into their lives by trying more of the dinners. Once you learn the calorie counts for your favorite snacks, it's really not that hard to count calories.

Table 15.3 supplies an alternative to counting calories. Any non-food group restricting diet plan that has you count, is counting calories. It may look like you're counting something else, but the underlying goal is restriction of calories by counting something.

The sizes of the food group servings are also based on average calories. If you learn what constitutes a serving, you can count food group servings.

The remainder of the book contains practical applications for the theories and concepts we've been discussing — shopping lists, menus and recipes. Before you start, do one last reality check. Have you picked a weight you can live with when you get there? Look at the number of calories that will sustain your goal weight and make sure it's a reasonable number. You're going to be eating it today, and tomorrow. In order to achieve and maintain the weight you've selected, you need to be happy eating this number of calories forever.

Every marathon starts with a first step. The loss of 100 pounds starts with losing a single pound. Good luck.

Part Two

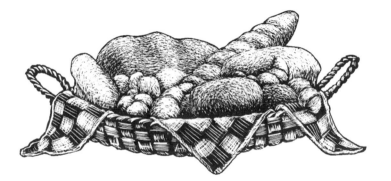

The Program

Grocery List
Week 1

Breads/Grains

Bagel. everything

Bagel, plain

French roll

Pita bread

Pancakes, low fat

Basmati rice

Linguine

Macaroni

Orzo pasta

Cornmeal, yellow

Granola cereal

Old-fashioned rolled oats

Oatmeal, instant (flavored)

White sandwich bread

Condiments

Allspice, ground

Apple cider vinegar

Baking powder

Baking soda

Barbecue sauce

Basil leaf, dried

Black pepper

Brown sugar

Canola oil

Cayenne pepper

Celery seed

Chili powder

Chocolate chips, semi-sweet

Cinnamon, ground

Cocoa powder, unsweetened

Cooking spray

Coriander seed, ground

Cumin seed, ground

Cumin seed, whole

Curry powder

Dijon mustard

Dill pickle relish

Dry mustard

Fennel seed, whole

Garlic powder, granulated

Granulated sugar

Honey

Iodized salt

Jalapeno peppers, pickled

Kosher salt

Lemon pepper

Mayonnaise, reduced fat

Nutella® chocolate hazelnut spread

Olive oil

Onion powder, granulated

Oregano, dried

Parsley flakes, dried

Peanut oil

Ranch dressing mix

Grocery List

Week 1

Red wine vinegar
Red pepper, crushed flakes
Sweet paprika
Sweet pickle relish
Syrup, blueberry-flavored
White wine vinegar
Worcestershire sauce
Yellow mustard

Dairy

Brie
Butter, unsalted
Buttermilk, 1%
Cheddar cheese
Egg substitute, liquid
Eggs, large
Feta cheese
Milk, skim
Smoked salmon cream cheese, light
Sour cream, light
Vanilla yogurt, fat free

Fruits

Blueberries
Granny Smith apples
Kiwifruit
Mango
Oranges

Papaya
Pineapple
Raisins
Raspberries
Strawberries

Meats

Canadian bacon
Chicken breast filets,
    boneless, skinless
Clams, canned, chopped
Ground beef, 96% extra lean
Honey ham, lean deli
Pork loin, center-cut
Salmon filets
Tuna, canned, solid white
    albacore in water

Vegetables

Asparagus
Bell peppers, yellow, red, and green
Carrots
Celery
Cherry tomatoes
Coleslaw mix, shredded
Corn, frozen, whole kernel
Cucumber
Fennel bulb

Grocery List
Week 1

Garlic

Green beans, frozen

Mushrooms, button

Onion, red

Onion, yellow

Parsley

Potatoes, fingerling

Potatoes, frozen, shredded

Potatoes, red

Potatoes, Russet or Idaho

Romaine lettuce

Roma tomatoes

Scallions

Spinach, fresh baby

Other

Almonds, slivered

Apple Spice Scrumpet™ mix

Beef broth, low fat

Chicken broth, fat free

Clam juice

Crackers, butter-flavored

Crushed tomatoes

Diced tomatoes in sauce

Doritos® chips, WOW™

Hummus, prepared

Kidney beans, canned

Olives, black

Petite diced tomatoes

Potato chips, fat free

Pretzels, fat free

Tomato paste

Tomato sauce

Tostidos® chips, WOW™

Day One

Breakfast
280 Calories, 4 grams of Fat

3/4 cup fat free vanilla yogurt

1 ounce granola cereal

1/2 cup fresh raspberries

Snack
150 Calories

Choose from snack list

Lunch
440 Calories, 11 grams of Fat

2 ounces lean deli honey ham and 1 ounce brie

2 ounce French roll

1 ounce fat free potato chips

small (3 ounce) Granny Smith apple

Dinner
510 Calories, 8.5 grams of Fat

Honey Mustard Chicken

Orzo Pilaf

Roasted Asparagus

1 cup skim milk

Snack
220 Calories

Choose from snack list

Bolded food items can be found in the recipe section of this book

Eucalorics

Day Two

Breakfast
290 Calories, 7 grams of Fat

3 ounce everything bagel

2 tablespoons light smoked salmon cream cheese

Snack
150 Calories

Choose from snack list

Lunch
420 Calories, 13 grams of Fat

Barbecue Ranch Chicken Salad

5 butter-flavored crackers

Dinner
500 Calories, 9 grams of Fat

Meatloaf

Buttermilk Mashed Potatoes

Country Green Beans

1 cup skim milk

Snack
240 Calories

Choose from snack list

Bolded food items can be found in the recipe section of this book

Day Three

Breakfast
320 Calories, 2.5 grams of Fat

3 low fat pancakes

2 tablespoons blueberry-flavored syrup

1/4 cup fresh blueberries

Snack
150 Calories

Choose from snack list

Lunch
410 Calories, 7 grams of Fat

Egg Salad

2 ounces white bread

1 ounce fat free pretzels

1 cup sliced strawberries with 1 medium (3 ounce) kiwifruit

Dinner
505 Calories, 11.5 grams of Fat

Linguine with White Clam Sauce

Rainbow Carrot and Pepper Sauté

1 cup skim milk

Snack
215 Calories

Choose from snack list

Bolded food items can be found in the recipe section of this book

Eucalorics

Day Four

Breakfast
250 Calories, 2 grams of Fat

1 ounce package flavored instant oatmeal

1 cup skim milk

Snack
150 Calories

Choose from snack list

Lunch
430 Calories, 9 grams of Fat

Tuna Grinder

1 ounce WOW™ Doritos® chips,

small (5 ounce) orange

Dinner
575 Calories, 14.5 grams of Fat

Tamale Pie with Cornbread Crust

Tossed Garden Salad with 2 tablespoons Ranch Dressing

1 cup skim milk

Snack
195 Calories

Choose from snack list

Bolded food items can be found in the recipe section of this book

Day Five

Breakfast

280 Calories, 10.5 grams of Fat

Bacon and Cheddar Omelet

Hash Brown Potatoes

Snack

150 Calories

Choose from snack list

Lunch

420 Calories, 9 grams of Fat

Caribbean Curried Chicken Salad

1 ounce pita bread

1/2 cup pineapple, 1/2 cup mango, and 1/2 cup papaya chunks

Dinner

500 Calories, 12.5 grams of Fat

Barbecue Rubbed Pork Loin

Mustard Potato Salad

Creamy Coleslaw

1 cup skim milk

Snack

250 Calories

Choose from snack list

Bolded food items can be found in the recipe section of this book

Eucalorics

Day Six

Breakfast

295 Calories, 4 grams of Fat

Chocolate Chocolate Chip Muffin

1 cup skim milk

Snack

150 Calories

Choose from snack list

Lunch

450 Calories, 20 grams of Fat

1/2 cup prepared hummus

1 ounce pita bread

Greek Cucumber and Tomato Salad

Dinner

475 Calories, 15 grams of Fat

Chicken Cacciatore

Tossed Garden Salad with Creamy Italian Dressing

Snack

230 Calories

Choose from snack list

Bolded food items can be found in the recipe section of this book

Day Seven

Breakfast

295 Calories, 4 grams of Fat

Apple Spice Scrumpet™ (prepared according to mix)

1 cup skim milk

Snack

150 Calories

Choose from snack list

Lunch

480 Calories, 9 grams of Fat

Beef and Bean Chili

1/2 ounce shredded cheddar cheese

chopped onion, chopped tomato and jalapeno pepper rings

1 ounce WOW™ Tostidos® chips

Dinner

425 Calories, 12.5 grams of Fat

Spice Crusted Salmon Filets

Roasted Fingerling Potatoes and Fennel

Sautéed Spinach with Onion

Snack

250 Calories

Choose from snack list

Bolded food items can be found in the recipe section of this book

Eucalorics

Grocery List
Week 2

Breads/Grains

Baguette

Basmati rice

Capellini (angel hair) pasta

Cold cereal, no nuts

Egg noodles, wide

English muffin, cinnamon raisin

Flour tortillas

Orzo pasta

Pumpernickel bread

Sourdough bread

White sandwich bread

Whole wheat roll

Wild rice, quick-cook/parboiled

Condiments

Anchovy paste

Bay leaves

Chipotle peppers in adobo sauce

Corn syrup, light

Garlic, minced dehydrated

Ketchup

Major Grey's chutney

Nutmeg, ground

Onion flakes, dehydrated

Thyme, dried

White pepper, ground

Dairy

American cheese, 2%

Blue cheese

Butter, unsalted

Buttermilk, 1%

Cojack cheese

Cottage cheese, low fat

Cream, heavy

Egg substitute, liquid

Eggs, large

Gruyere cheese

Milk, skim

Parmesan cheese

Sour cream, light

Swiss cheese, baby

Fruits

Apple

Banana

Cantaloupe

Cranberries, sweetened, dried

Grapes, red

Honeydew melon

Lemons

Nectarine

Peaches, canned in juice

Pineapple

Grocery List

Week 2

Meats

Andouille sausage
Bacon
Canadian bacon
Chicken breast filets,
    boneless, skinless
Corned beef, lean deli
Ground beef, 96% extra lean
Honey ham, lean deli
Pollack, filets
Pork loin, center-cut
Roast beef, lean deli
Shrimp, cooked, peeled large
Shrimp, cooked, baby salad
Turkey breast, lean deli smoked

Vegetables

Bell pepper, green and red
Broccoli florettes
Carrots, baby
Celery
Cherry tomatoes
Corn, frozen, whole kernel
Garlic
Green beans, fresh
Onion, yellow
Leek
Mushrooms, button

Mushrooms, dehydrated exotic
    (chanterelles, porcinis, or
    shitakes)
Okra, frozen
Parsley
Potatoes, Yukon gold
Roma tomatoes
Romaine lettuce
Scallions
Thyme, fresh
Tomatoes
Zucchini

Other

Beef broth, low fat
Black beans, canned
Cherry Almond Scrumpet™ mix
Chicken broth, fat free
Clam juice
Cream of mushroom soup
Diced tomatoes
Green chilies, mild, canned
Kidney beans, canned
Melba toast, rounds
Onion soup mix, dry
Peanut butter
Pecan pieces
Potato chips, Lays®, WOW™
Pretzels, fat free

Red wine
Saltines
Sauerkraut
Strawberry jam, sugar-free
Sour cream and onion
      potato chips, WOW™
Tomato juice
Tomato paste
Vegetable stock

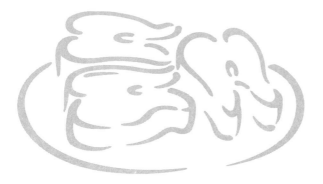

Day Eight

Breakfast
235 Calories, 2 grams of Fat

1 ounce cold cereal (no nuts)

1/2 cup skim milk

1 medium (5 ounce) banana

Snack
150 Calories

Choose from snack list

Lunch
460 Calories, 14 grams of Fat

2 ounces lean deli smoked turkey breast and 1 ounce cojack cheese

2 ounces sourdough bread

1 tablespoon reduced fat mayonnaise with 1/4 teaspoon chili powder,

1/8 teaspoon ground cumin seed, pinch kosher salt and black pepper

1 ounce WOW™ Sour Cream and Onion potato chips

1 medium (4 ounce) nectarine

Dinner
515 Calories, 10.5 grams of Fat

Garlic and Pepper Crusted Pork Loin

Cranberry Wild Rice

Glazed Carrots

1 cup skim milk

Snack
240 Calories

Choose from snack list

Bolded food items can be found in the recipe section of this book

Eucalorics

Day Nine

Breakfast

350 Calories, 8.5 grams of Fat

1 cinnamon raisin English muffin

1/2 tablespoon unsalted butter

1 large (8 ounce) apple

Snack

150 Calories

Choose from snack list

Lunch

405 Calories, 15.5 grams of Fat

Cobb Salad

6 saltine crackers

Dinner

495 Calories, 10 grams of Fat

Ground Beef Stroganoff with Buttered Egg Noodles

Sautéed Green Beans with Carrots and Bell Peppers

1 cup skim milk

Snack

200 Calories

Choose from snack list

Bolded food items can be found in the recipe section of this book

Day Ten

Breakfast

275 Calories, 12 grams of Fat

Vegetable Frittata

1/2 cup honeydew and 1/2 cup cantaloupe

Snack

150 Calories

Choose from snack list

Lunch

450 Calories, 8 grams of Fat

Mango Ginger Curried Shrimp Salad

1 ounce melba toast rounds

Dinner

475 Calories, 12.5 grams of Fat

Mushroom Smothered Chicken

Garlic Mashed Potatoes

Zucchini with Leeks

1 cup skim milk

Snack

250 Calories

Choose from snack list

Bolded food items can be found in the recipe section of this book

Day Eleven

Breakfast

220 Calories, 3 grams of Fat

1 cup low fat cottage cheese

1/2 cup canned peaches, in juice

Snack

150 Calories

Choose from snack list

Lunch

490 Calories, 15.5 grams of Fat

2 ounces pumpernickel bread

2 ounces lean deli corned beef

1 ounce baby Swiss cheese

2 tablespoons Thousand Island Dressing

2 tablespoons sauerkraut

1 ounce fat free pretzel twists

Dinner

535 Calories, 11.5 grams of Fat

Black Pepper and Parmesan Shrimp Capellini

Tossed Garden Salad with 2 tablespoons Green Goddess Dressing

1 cup skim milk

Snack

205 Calories

Choose from snack list

Bolded food items can be found in the recipe section of this book

Day Twelve

Breakfast

245 Calories, 10 grams of Fat

2 ounces sliced white bread, toasted

1 tablespoon peanut butter

1 tablespoon sugar-free strawberry jam

Snack

150 Calories

Choose from snack list

Lunch

465 Calories, 10.5 grams of Fat

Honey Pecan Chicken Salad

2 ounce wheat roll

1 cup red grapes

Dinner

510 Calories, 10.5 grams of Fat

Cajun Pork Roast

Red Beans and Rice

Tomatoes and Okra

1 cup skim milk

Snack

230 Calories

Choose from snack list

Bolded food items can be found in the recipe section of this book

Day Thirteen

Breakfast

Banana Muffin

1 cup skim milk

Snack

150 Calories

Choose from snack list

Lunch

480 Calories, 10 grams of Fat

2 ounce tortilla

1 ounce lean deli honey ham

1 ounce lean deli smoked turkey

1 ounce lean deli roast beef

1 slice 2% American cheese

1 ounce WOW™ Lays® Potato Chips

1 cup pineapple chunks

Dinner

465 Calories, 11 grams of Fat

Chipotle Chicken

Mexican Corn and Black Beans

Tossed Salad with 1/2 ounce Monterey Jack Cheese and

2 tablespoons Chipotle Ranch Dressing

Snack

215 Calories

Choose from snack list

Bolded food items can be found in the recipe section of this book

Day Fourteen

Breakfast
295 Calories, 4 grams of Fat

Cherry Almond Scrumpet™ (prepared according to mix)

1 cup skim milk

Snack
150 Calories

Choose from snack list

Lunch
425 Calories, 15 grams of Fat

Forest Mushroom Soup

Swiss Toast

Dinner
510 Calories, 9 grams of Fat

Lemon Pollock

Ham and Parmesan Orzo

Garlic Broccoli

1 cup skim milk

Snack
220 Calories

Choose from snack list

Bolded food items can be found in the recipe section of this book

Grocery List
Week 3

Breads/Grains

Arborio rice
Bagel, blueberry
Bagel, plain
Basmati rice
Blueberry bagel
Bread cubes, dry, unseasoned
Cold cereal, no nuts
Cream of Wheat, instant
English muffin, plain
Flour tortillas
French roll
Italian roll
Macaroni
Orzo pasta
Penne
Rye bread

Condiments/Seasonings

Chives, freeze-dried
Hot sauce
Mustard, spicy brown
Old Bay seasoning
Poultry seasoning
Sage, rubbed
Salsa
Sweet pickles

Dairy

American cheese, 2%
Butter, unsalted
Cheddar cheese
Cream, heavy
Flounder filets
Gruyere cheese
Egg substitute, liquid
Milk, skim
Milk, whole
Mexican-blend cheese, shredded
Mozzarella cheese, part-skim
Parmesan cheese
Sour cream, light
Strawberry cream cheese, light
Swiss cheese, baby

Fruits

Apples, frozen without sugar
Apple, Granny Smith
Banana
Cantaloupe
Grapefruit
Grapes, green
Honeydew melon
Lemon
Orange
Pear

Grocery List
Week 3

Meats

Andouille sausage

Chicken breast filets,
    boneless, skinless

Crabmeat, imitation

Crabmeat, cooked lump

Crawfish tailmeat, cooked

Ground beef, 96% extra lean

Pastrami, lean deli

Pork loin, center-cut

Vegetables

Asparagus

Bell pepper, green and red

Broccoli florettes

Carrots, baby

Cauliflower florettes

Celery

Cherry tomatoes

Corn, frozen, whole kernel

Green beans, fresh

Garlic

Onion, red

Onion, yellow

Mushrooms, button

Parsley

Potatoes, Russet or Idaho

Roma tomatoes

Romaine lettuce

Scallions

Sugar snap peas, fresh

Tarragon, fresh

Zucchini

Other

Beef broth, low fat

Chicken broth, fat free

Cracker crumbs

Crushed tomatoes

Diced tomatoes

Lemon Blueberry Scrumpet™ mix

Potato chips, Ruffles®, WOW®

Refried beans, fat free

Sherry wine, dry

Tarragon vinegar

Tomato sauce

Vegetable broth

Walnut pieces

White wine

Eucalorics

Day Fifteen

Breakfast

235 Calories, 2 grams of Fat

1 ounce cold cereal (no nuts)

1/2 cup skim milk

1 medium (5 ounce) banana

Snack

150 Calories

Choose from snack list

Lunch

440 Calories, 14 grams of Fat

2 ounces rye bread

2 ounces lean deli pastrami

1 ounce baby Swiss cheese

1 tablespoon spicy brown mustard

1 ounce WOW® Ruffles® potato chips

Dinner

575 Calories, 12.5 grams of Fat

Chili Mac

Tossed Garden Salad with 2 tablespoons Thousand Island Dressing

1 cup skim milk

Snack

200 Calories

Choose from snack list

Bolded food items can be found in the recipe section of this book

Day Sixteen

Breakfast

290 Calories, 6.5 grams of Fat

3 ounce blueberry bagel

2 tablespoons light strawberry cream cheese

Snack

150 Calories

Choose from snack list

Lunch

395 Calories, 11.5 grams of Fat

Chicken Caesar Salad

2 ounce sourdough roll

Dinner

530 Calories, 11.5 grams of Fat

Roasted Pork Loin with Mushroom Stuffing

Cinnamon Apples

1 cup skim milk

Snack

235 Calories

Choose from snack list

Bolded food items can be found in the recipe section of this book

Eucalorics

Day Seventeen

Breakfast
320 Calories, 7 grams of Fat

3 ounce plain bagel toasted with **Cinnamon Sugar Spread**

Snack
150 Calories

Choose from snack list

Lunch
400 Calories, 9 grams of Fat

Corn and Crab Pasta Salad

1 cup green grapes

Dinner
490 Calories, 13 grams of Fat

Chicken and Mushroom Risotto

California Medley

1 cup skim milk

Snack
205 Calories

Choose from snack list

Bolded food items can be found in the recipe section of this book

Day Eighteen

Breakfast
275 Calories, 0 grams of Fat

1 ounce package instant Cream of Wheat

1/2 large (1 pound) grapefruit with 1 tablespoon sugar

1 cup skim milk

Snack
150 Calories

Choose from snack list

Lunch
410 Calories, 14.5 grams of Fat

Italian Ham and Mozzarella Melt

1/2 cup honeydew and 1/2 cup cantaloupe

Dinner
565 Calories, 9 grams of Fat

Spaghetti with Meat Sauce

Tossed Salad with 2 tablespoons Creamy Italian Dressing

1 cup skim milk

Snack
215 Calories

Choose from snack list

Bolded food items can be found in the recipe section of this book

Eucalorics

Day Nineteen

Breakfast

265 Calories, 5.5 grams of Fat

Huevos Rancheros

1 medium (7 ounce) orange

Snack

150 Calories

Choose from snack list

Lunch

415 Calories, 14 grams of Fat

Tarragon Chicken Salad

2 ounce french roll

Marinated Asparagus

Dinner

480 Calories, 12.5 grams of Fat

Andouille and Crawfish Trinity

Scallion and Parsley Pilaf

Garlic Zucchini

1 cup skim milk

Snack

290 Calories

Choose from snack list

Bolded food items can be found in the recipe section of this book

Day Twenty

Breakfast

255 Calories, 4 grams of Fat

Breakfast Sandwich

1 medium (3 ounce) plum

Snack

150 Calories

Choose from snack list

Lunch

465 Calories, 14 grams of Fat

Soft Bean Burritos

1/2 cup papaya chunks

Dinner

520 Calories, 8 grams of Fat

Barbecue Chicken

Cheddar and Chive Mashed Potatoes

Green Beans with Red Onion and Red Pepper

1 cup skim milk

Snack

210 Calories

Choose from snack list

Bolded food items can be found in the recipe section of this book

Eucalorics

Day Twenty-One

Breakfast

295 Calories, 4 grams of Fat

Lemon Blueberry Scrumpet™ (prepared according to mix)

1 cup skim milk

Snack

150 Calories

Choose from snack list

Lunch

420 Calories, 11 grams of Fat

Cream of Chicken Corn Soup

Cornbread

1 medium (6 ounce) pear

Dinner

535 Calories, 13 grams of Fat

Stuffed Flounder

Lemon Pepper Orzo

Buttered Sugar Snap Peas

1 cup skim milk

Snack

200 Calories

Choose from snack list

Bolded food items can be found in the recipe section of this book

Grocery List
Week 4

Breads/Grains
Basmati rice
Buttermilk biscuits,
    Pillsbury, 7.5-ounce can
Cold cereal, no nuts
Couscous
Egg noodles
Flour tortillas
Focaccia, plain
Grits, instant
Hamburger buns
Macaroni
Orzo pasta
Pearled barley
Sourdough roll
Waffles, fat free, frozen
Whole wheat sandwich bread

Condiments/Seasonings
Apple butter
Distilled wine vinegar
Maple syrup
Rice wine, Japanese (mirin)
Rosemary, dried
Seasoned rice vinegar
Soy sauce, low sodium
Toasted sesame oil

Dairy
Butter, unsalted
Buttermilk, 1%
Cheddar cheese
Egg substitute, liquid
Eggs, large
Mexican-cheese, shredded
Milk, skim
Parmesan cheese
Pecorino cheese
Sour cream, light
Velveeta cheese®, light

Fruits
Banana
Currants
Grapes, red
Honeydew melon
Lemon
Lime
Mandarin orange segments,
    canned in juice
Strawberries

Meats
Andouille sausage
Cod filets
Chicken breast filets,
    boneless, skinless

Grocery List
Week 4

Country ham
Ground beef, 96% extra lean
Pork loin, center-cut
Roast beef, lean deli
Tuna, canned,
      solid white albacore in water

Vegetables
Bell pepper, green & red
Carrots, baby
Carrots and peas, frozen
Cauliflower florettes
Celery
Cherry tomatoes
Cilantro, fresh
Coleslaw mix, shredded
Garlic
Ginger, fresh
Green beans, fresh
Green beans, frozen
Mint, fresh
Mushrooms, button
Onion, red
Onion, yellow
Parsley
Peas, frozen
Potatoes, new
Romaine lettuce
Rosemary, fresh

Scallions
Seaphire
Sugar snap peas, fresh
Thyme, fresh
Tomato
Tomatoes, sun dried
Zucchini

Other
Almonds, sliced
Beef broth, low fat
Chicken broth, fat free
Cream of mushroom soup
Cornstarch
Diced tomatoes
Great Northern beans, canned
Green chilies, mild, canned
Orange Cranberry Scrumpet™ mix
Potato chips, WOW™ barbecue
Potato chips, Ruffles®, WOW®
Sesame crackers
Tomato juice
Tomato sauce
Vegetable broth

Day Twenty-Two

Breakfast
235 Calories, 2 grams of Fat

1 ounce cold cereal (no nuts)

1/2 cup skim milk

1 medium (5 ounce) banana

Snack
150 Calories

Choose from snack list

Lunch
465 Calories, 14.5 grams of Fat

2 ounces lean deli roast beef

1 ounce cheddar cheese

1 tablespoon reduced fat mayonnaise

1 ounce WOW® Barbecue potato chips

1 cup fresh strawberries, sliced

Dinner
505 Calories, 9 grams of Fat

Chili Stuffed Pepper

Mexican Rice

Zucchini with Tomatoes and Cumin

1 cup skim milk

Snack
245 Calories

Choose from snack list

Bolded food items can be found in the recipe section of this book

Eucalorics

Day Twenty-Three

Breakfast
275 Calories, 7 grams of Fat

Cinnamon Raisin Pull-Apart

1 cup fresh strawberries

Snack
150 Calories

Choose from snack list

Lunch
415 calories, 4 grams of Fat

Sloppy Joes

1 ounce WOW® Ruffles® potato chips

1 cup red grapes

Dinner
510 Calories, 9.5 grams of Fat

Onion and Rosemary Chicken

Couscous with Currants

Buttered Cauliflower

1 cup skim milk

Snack
200 Calories

Choose from snack list

Bolded food items can be found in the recipe section of this book

Day Twenty-Four

Breakfast
290 Calories, 0 grams of Fat

2 fat free frozen waffles

2 tablespoons maple syrup

1 cup honeydew

Snack
150 Calories

Choose from snack list

Lunch
475 Calories, 25 grams of Fat

Mandarin Chicken Salad with Asian Vinaigrette

6 sesame crackers

Dinner
465 Calories, 16 grams of Fat

Italian Seasoned Pork Loin

Orzo Primavera

Sugar Snap Pea and Pecorino Salad

Snack
220 Calories

Choose from snack list

Bolded food items can be found in the recipe section of this book

Eucalorics

Day Twenty-Five

Breakfast

235 Calories, 2 grams of Fat

1 ounce cold cereal (no nuts)

1/2 cup skim milk

1 medium (5 ounce) banana

Snack

150 Calories

Choose from snack list

Lunch

480 Calories, 17.5 grams of Fat

Open-Faced Chicken Quesadillas

Fresh Tomato Salsa

Dinner

490 Calories, 12 grams of Fat

Tuna Noodle Casserole

2/3 cup prepared frozen carrots and peas

Snack

245 Calories

Choose from snack list

Bolded food items can be found in the recipe section of this book

Day Twenty-Six

Breakfast
265 Calories, 9 grams of Fat

Cheddar Grits

1 large (6 ounce) peach

Snack
150 Calories

Choose from snack list

Lunch
420 Calories, 6 grams of Fat

Tuna Salad

2 ounces whole wheat bread

1 ounce WOW™ Lays® potato chips

1 medium (6 ounce) pear

Dinner
490 Calories, 8 grams of Fat

Teriyaki Chicken

Vegetable Lo Mein

Spicy Green Beans

Snack
270 Calories

Choose from snack list

Bolded food items can be found in the recipe section of this book

Day Twenty-Seven

Breakfast
290 Calories, 4 grams of Fat

Orange Cranberry Scrumpet™ (prepared according to mix)

1 cup skim milk

Snack
150 Calories

Choose from snack list

Lunch
445 Calories, 8.5 grams of Fat

Minestrone

Sun Dried Tomato and Parmesan Focaccia

Dinner
490 Calories, 11 grams of Fat

Rosemary and Thyme Pork Loin

Barley Pilaf

Buttered Carrots

1 cup skim milk

Snack
225 Calories

Choose from snack list

Bolded food items can be found in the recipe section of this book

Day Twenty-Eight

Breakfast

295 Calories, 4 grams of Fat

Brown Sugar Apple Butter Muffin

1 cup skim milk

Snack

150 Calories

Choose from snack list

Lunch

390 Calories, 10 grams of Fat

Cajun Chicken Salad

2 ounce sourdough roll

1 cup cherry tomatoes

Dinner

515 Calories, 11 grams of Fat

Mustard and Cheese Cod

Buttered and Parsley New Potatoes

Roasted Seaphire

1 cup skim milk

Snack

250 Calories

Choose from snack list

Bolded food items can be found in the recipe section of this book

Eucalorics

Bacon and Cheddar Omelet

1 Portion • 180 Calories, 6 grams of Fat

3/4 cup	liquid egg substitute
1 ounce	Canadian bacon, diced
1/2 ounce	cheddar cheese, shredded
	kosher salt
	ground black pepper
	cooking spray

Coat a nonstick omelet pan or small skillet with cooking spray and place over medium high heat. Season the egg substitute with salt and pepper. When the pan is hot, pour the egg substitute into the pan, and cook without stirring until the omelet begins to set and bubble up around the edges, about 15 seconds. With a spatula, lift up the edge of the omelet to allow the still liquid egg to run beneath it. Continue until the bottom of the omelet is set, about 1 minute. Top the omelet with the bacon and cheese. Using the spatula, fold half of the omelet onto itself. Cook 1 minute more, until the omelet is cooked through. Invert the omelet onto a plate.

Breakfast

Hash Brown Potatoes

1 Portion • 100 Calories, 4.5 grams of Fat

1/2 cup	fresh or frozen peeled and shredded potatoes
1 tsp	peanut oil
1/8 tsp	kosher salt
	black pepper

Preheat oven to 300 degrees. Heat oil in a nonstick skillet over high heat until almost smoking. Add potatoes, salt, and pepper. Cook, stirring frequently, until the potatoes are nicely browned, 4-5 minutes. Place in the oven to keep warm while preparing the Bacon and Cheddar Omelet.

Chocolate Chocolate Chip Muffins

6 Portions • 205 Calories, 4.5 grams of Fat

2 tbsps	Nutella® Chocolate Hazelnut Spread
1/2 cup	granulated sugar
1/2 cup	liquid egg substitute
2/3 cup	all-purpose flour
1/3 cup	unsweetened cocoa powder
1/2 tsp	baking soda
1/8 tsp	iodized salt
1/2 cup	1% buttermilk
1/4 cup	semi-sweet chocolate chips

Preheat oven to 350 degrees. Cream together Nutella® and sugar. Stir in the egg substitute and beat until smooth. Stir together the flour, cocoa, soda and salt. Alternate adding the cocoa mixture and buttermilk, beginning and ending with the cocoa. Fold in the chocolate chips. Line a 6-cup muffin pan with paper liners. Divide batter between the 6 muffin cups. Bake for 22-25 minutes, until a tester comes out of the center clean and the top of the muffin springs back if pressed.

Helpful Tips

Out of buttermilk? Substitute 1/2 cup skim milk mixed with 1/2 tbsp white vinegar.

Vegetable Frittata

1 Portion • 215 Calories, 12 grams of Fat

3/4 cup	liquid egg substitute
1 tsp	olive oil
2 tbsps	yellow onion, finely chopped (.5 ounces)
2 tbsps	green bell pepper, finely chopped (.5 ounces)
1 ounce	button mushrooms, sliced
1	Roma tomato, diced
1/2 ounce	Parmesan cheese, finely grated
	pinch dried basil leaf
	pinch granulated garlic powder
	pinch kosher salt
	pinch black pepper

Preheat oven to 350 degrees. Heat the oil in a small, nonstick skillet over medium high heat. Sauté the onion and bell pepper until the onions and peppers begin to color, 3-4 minutes. Stir in the tomatoes and mushrooms and cook an additional minute. In a bowl whisk together the egg, basil, garlic, salt and pepper. Pour over the vegetable mixture. Cook for 2-3 minutes until it begins to set. Sprinkle the top with the Parmesan cheese and place in the oven. Bake for 8-10 minutes, until the frittata is cooked through and the cheese has melted.

Banana Muffin

6 Portions • 200 Calories, 4 grams of Fat

2 tbsps	unsalted butter, softened
1/2 cup	granulated sugar
1/2 cup	liquid egg substitute
1/2 cup	ripe banana, mashed
1 cup	all-purpose flour
1/2 tsp	baking soda
1/8 tsp	iodized salt
1/2 cup	1% buttermilk

Preheat oven to 350 degrees. Cream together the butter and sugar. Stir in the egg substitute and banana and beat until smooth. Stir together the flour, soda and salt. Alternate adding the flour mixture and buttermilk, beginning and ending with the flour. Line a 6-cup muffin pan with paper liners. Divide batter between the 6 muffin cups. Bake for 22-25 minutes, until a tester comes out of the center clean and the top of the muffin springs back if pressed.

Helpful Tips

Don't put your overripe bananas in the garbage. Instead, freeze them in their skin until the next time you make banana muffins.

Cinnamon Sugar Spread

1 Portion • 100 Calories, 5.5 grams of Fat

1/2 tbsp	unsalted butter, softened
1 tbsp	brown sugar (packed)
1/8 tsp	ground cinnamon

Combine butter, sugar and cinnamon until a smooth spread is achieved. Use spread to top bagels, bread or English muffins before toasting.

Huevos Rancheros

1 Portion • 195 Calories, 6 grams of Fat

1	1-ounce flour tortilla
1/2 cup	liquid egg substitute
1/2 ounce	Mexican-blend cheese, shredded
2 tbsps	salsa
	cooking spray

Coat a small nonstick skillet with cooking spray and heat over medium high heat. When the pan is hot, add the eggs and scramble until cooked through. Place in the center of the tortilla and top with cheese and salsa, before rolling like a burrito.

Breakfast Sandwich

1 Portion • 210 Calories, 4 grams of Fat

1	plain English muffin
1/4 cup	liquid egg substitute
1 slice	2% American cheese
	pinch kosher salt
	pinch black pepper
	cooking spray

Toast the English muffin. Coat a small nonstick skillet with cooking spray. Season the egg substitute with salt and pepper, then scramble over medium heat until cooked through. Mound the eggs in the center and top with the cheese. Allow to cook for 2-3 minutes over low heat, until the cheese is melted. Place the egg on half the English muffin and top with the other half.

Cinnamon Raisin Pull-Aparts

5 Portions • 215 Calories, 6 grams of Fat

1	can Pillsbury buttermilk biscuits (7.5-ounce size)
2 tbsp	unsalted butter, melted
1/3 cup	brown sugar, packed
1/2 tsp	ground cinnamon
2 tbsps	raisins
	cooking spray

Preheat the oven to 350 degrees. Coat a 6-cup muffin pan with cooking spray. Combine the cinnamon and sugar. Cut each biscuit in half and roll it into a ball. Dip the balls in butter, then roll in the cinnamon sugar. Place 4 balls in each muffin cup. Sprinkle each cup with 1 teaspoon of raisins. Bake for 15-17 minutes, until the biscuits are cooked through.

Cheddar Grits

1 Portion • 210 Calories, 9 grams of Fat

1	packet instant Grits (1-ounce package)
1 ounce	shredded cheddar cheese
	pinch kosher salt
	pinch black pepper
	pinch granulated garlic powder

Prepare grits as the package directs. Stir in cheese, heating if necessary to fully melt it. Stir in a pinch of kosher salt, black pepper and granulated garlic.

Brown Sugar Apple Butter Muffins

6 Portions • 205 Calories, 4 grams of Fat

2 tbsps	unsalted butter, softened
1/2 cup	brown sugar, packed
1/2 cup	liquid egg substitute
1/2 cup	apple butter
1 cup	all-purpose flour
1/2 tsp	baking soda
1/8 tsp	iodized salt
1/2 tsp	ground cinnamon
1/4 tsp	ground nutmeg
1/2 cup	1% buttermilk

Preheat oven to 350 degrees. Cream together the butter and sugar. Stir in the egg substitute and apple butter and beat until smooth. Stir together the flour, soda, salt, cinnamon and nutmeg. Alternate adding the flour mixture and buttermilk, beginning and ending with the flour. Line a 6-cup muffin pan with paper liners. Divide batter between the 6 muffin cups. Bake for 22-25 minutes, until a tester comes out of the center clean and the top of the muffin springs back if pressed.

Egg Salad

6 Portions • 100 Calories, 5 grams of Fat

9	large eggs, hardboiled
3 tbsps	yellow onion, finely chopped (1 ounce)
1/2 cup	celery, chopped (2 ounces)
1/2 cup	reduced fat mayonnaise
1 tbsp	yellow mustard
2 tbsps	dill pickle relish
1 tsp	granulated sugar
	kosher salt
	black pepper

Finely chop 3 whole hardboiled eggs and 6 hardboiled egg whites (discarding extra yolks). Add the onion and celery. In a small bowl combine mayonnaise, mustard, relish and sugar. Toss the dressing with the eggs. Season to taste with salt and pepper.

Helpful Tips

Eggs that are 1-2 weeks old peel easier than eggs that are fresh.

Barbecue Ranch Grilled Chicken Salad

1 Portion • 340 Calories, 9 grams of Fat

1	4-ounce boneless, skinless chicken breast filet
2 tbsps	homemade or store-bought barbecue sauce
4 ounces	romaine or other dark leafy lettuce
1/4 cup	scallions, sliced thin
1	Roma tomato, diced
1	large egg, hardboiled and grated
3 tbsps	Barbecue Ranch Dressing (below)

Coat chicken breast with barbecue sauce and grill or broil until cooked through, 6-8 minutes per side. Slice chicken into thin strips, then toss with lettuce, scallions, tomato and egg. Top with Barbecue Ranch Dressing.

Lunch

Barbecue Ranch Dressing

3 tbsp	Ranch Dressing (pg.229)
1 tbsp	homemade or store-bought barbecue sauce

Whisk together dressing and barbecue sauce. Refrigerate for at least 15 minutes before using.

1 Portion • 60 Calories, 2 grams of Fat

Eucalorics

Caribbean Curry Chicken Salad

6 Portions • 225 Calories, 8 grams of Fat

1 recipe	Poached Chicken for Salad (below)
3/4 cup	celery, diced (3 ounces)
1/4 cup	bell pepper, diced (1 ounce)
1/4 cup	scallions, sliced thin
1 clove	garlic, minced
1/3 cup	reduced fat mayonnaise
1/2 cup	light sour cream
1/4 cup	raisins
1 ounce	slivered almonds, toasted
1 1/2 tsps	curry powder
1/8 tsp	ground cinnamon
1/2 tsp	kosher salt
	pinch ground allspice
	(optional) pinch ground cayenne pepper

Combine the chicken, celery, bell peppers, scallions, raisins and almonds. In a small bowl mix together the garlic, mayonnaise, sour cream, curry powder, cinnamon, salt, allspice and cayenne pepper. Toss the chicken mixture with the curried dressing. Salad may be chilled several hours or served immediately.

Poached Chicken

1 1/2 lbs	boneless skinless chicken breast

Place chicken in a large saucepan and cover with cold water. Bring to a boil over high heat, then turn to low and simmer the chicken for 15-20 minutes, until cooked through. Cool to room temperature and cut or pull into bite-sized pieces.

6 Portions • 120 Calories, 2 grams of Fat

Tuna Grinder

1 Portions • 290 Calories, 8 grams of Fat

1/2	3-ounce plain bagel
1	can solid white albacore tuna,
	packed in water (3-ounce)
1 tbsp	reduced fat mayonnaise
	kosher salt
	ground black pepper
1/2 ounce	cheddar cheese, sliced

Preheat the broiler. Drain the tuna well, then break up chunks into small flakes with a fork. Stir in mayonnaise and season with salt and pepper. Spread the tuna mixture on top of the bagel half. Top with sliced cheddar cheese. Place the tuna grinder on a cookie sheet and place beneath the broiler. Broil for 5-7 minutes, until the cheese is melted and the bagel is brown around the edges.

Beef and Bean Chili

6 Portions • 335 Calories, 3.5 grams of Fat

1 lb	96% extra lean ground beef
1 cup	yellow onion, chopped (5.5 ounces)
2	cans kidney beans, rinsed and drained (15-ounces each)
1	can tomato sauce (29-ounce)
1	can crushed tomatoes (28-ounce)
1	can petite diced tomatoes (14.5-ounce)
2 cups	low fat beef broth
3 tbsps	chili powder
1 tsp	kosher salt
3/4 tsp	ground cumin seed
1/4 tsp	granulated garlic powder
1/4 tsp	dried oregano
1/4 tsp	crushed red pepper flakes
1/4 tsp	black pepper
1/8 tsp	cayenne pepper

In a large Dutch oven, brown the ground beef with the onion, stirring frequently to break up beef. When the beef is cooked through, add the beans, chili powder, salt, cumin, garlic powder, oregano, red pepper flakes, black pepper and cayenne pepper. Cook for 5 minutes, then stir in the crushed tomatoes, tomato sauce, diced tomatoes and beef broth. Allow to simmer 30-40 minutes before serving.

Lunch

Greek Tomato and Cucumber Salad

6 Portions • 90 Calories, 7.5 grams of Fat

1	large cucumber (8"), peeled and chunked
4	Roma tomatoes quartered and seeded
1/2 cup	green bell pepper, sliced (1.5 ounces)
1/2 cup	yellow onion, sliced (2 ounces)
6	medium black olives, sliced
2 ounces	feta cheese, crumbled
2 tbsps	olive oil
1 tbsp	red wine vinegar
1/4 tsp	dried oregano
1 clove	fresh garlic, minced
1/8 tsp	kosher salt
1/8 tsp	dried parsley flakes
	pinch black pepper

In a large bowl, whisk together the oil and vinegar, then stir in the oregano, garlic, salt, parsley and black pepper. Add vegetables and feta and toss until everything is well coated. Refrigerate and allow to rest for at least 15 minutes before serving.

Lunch

Mango Ginger Curried Shrimp Salad

2 Portions • 335 Calories, 6 grams of Fat

1 lb	cooked salad shrimp
3/4 cup	celery, diced (3 ounces)
1/4 cup	green bell pepper, diced (1 ounce)
1/4 cup	scallions, sliced thin
1/4 cup	reduced fat mayonnaise
1/4 cup	light sour cream
3 tbsps	Major Grey's chutney
1 1/2 tsps	curry powder
1/2 tsp	kosher salt
	Optional — pinch cayenne pepper

Combine shrimp, celery, bell pepper and scallions. In a small bowl combine mayonnaise, sour cream, chutney, curry powder, salt and cayenne pepper. Toss the shrimp with the curried dressing. Chill the salad several hours or serve immediately.

Cobb Salad

1 Portion • 345 Calories, 14.5 grams of Fat

1	4-ounce boneless, skinless chicken breast filet
1 ounce	Canadian bacon, diced
4 ounces	romaine or other dark leafy lettuce
1	Roma tomato, diced
1	large egg, hardboiled and grated
3 tbsps	Blue Cheese Dressing (below)

Grill or broil chicken until cooked through, 6-8 minutes per side. Slice chicken into thin strips, then toss with bacon, lettuce, tomato and egg. Top with Blue Cheese Dressing.

Blue Cheese Dressing

1/4 cup	reduced fat mayonnaise
1/4 cup	light sour cream
1/3 cup	skim milk
1 1/2 tsps	red wine vinegar
3 ounces	blue cheese, crumbled
1/2 tsp	dried parsley flakes
1/8 tsp	granulated garlic powder
2 dashes	Worcestershire sauce
	pinch kosher salt
	pinch black pepper

Combine mayonnaise, sour cream, milk, vinegar, 2 ounces blue cheese, parsley, garlic, Worcestershire, salt and pepper in a blender or food processor. Process until smooth. Fold in remaining ounce of blue cheese.

6-3 tbsps Portions • 85 Calories, 6 grams of Fat

Lunch

Eucalorics

Honey Pecan Chicken Salad

6 Portions • 215 Calories, 8.5 grams of Fat

1 Recipe	Poached Chicken for Salad (pg. 149)
1 cup	celery, diced (4 ounces)
1/4 cup	scallions, sliced thin
1/2 cup	reduced fat mayonnaise
1/4 cup	light sour cream
1 tsp	Dijon mustard
2 tbsps	honey, divided
1 ounce	pecan pieces
3/4 tsp	kosher salt
	pinch black pepper

In a small saucepan combine pecan pieces and 1 tbsp of honey. Cook over medium high heat until the pecans are well coated and are nicely toasted, about 5 minutes. Spray a pan with non-stick spray and place the nuts in a single layer. Allow them to cool, then break up any clumps that form. Mix the honeyed pecans with the chicken, celery and scallions. In a small bowl combine mayonnaise, Dijon mustard, remaining tbsp of honey, salt and pepper. Toss dressing with chicken mixture. Salad may be chilled several hours or served immediately.

Swiss Toast

6 Portions • 255 Calories, 9 grams of Fat

1	**12-ounce baguette**
6 ounces	**gruyere cheese, grated**
	ground nutmeg

Preheat the broiler. Split the baguette lengthwise. Divide the cheese between each half. Sprinkle lightly with nutmeg. Place under broiler and toast until the cheese is completely melted and begins to brown around the edges.

Lunch

Grilled Chicken Caesar Salad

1 Portion • 245 Calories, 9.5 grams of Fat

1	4-ounce boneless, skinless chicken breast filet
4 ounces	romaine lettuce
3 tbsps	Caesar Dressing (below)
1/2 ounce	Parmesan cheese, finely shredded

Grill or broil chicken until cooked through, 6-8 minutes per side. Toss lettuce with dressing until well coated. Slice chicken into thin strips and top lettuce with it and Parmesan cheese.

Caesar Dressing

1/3 cup	reduced fat mayonnaise
1/4 cup	light sour cream
1/2 cup	skim milk
1 tbsp	fresh lemon juice
3 cloves	garlic, mashed to a paste
1 tsp	anchovy paste
1/4 tsp	kosher salt
1/2 tsp	black pepper
2 ounces	Parmesan cheese, finely grated

Combine all ingredients. Refrigerate at least 15 minutes before using. Caesar dressing will keep 2-3 days in the refrigerator.

8 – 3 tbsps Portions • 65 Calories, 4 grams of Fat

Lunch

Forest Mushroom Soup

6 Portions • 170 Calories, 8 grams of Fat

1 ounce	bacon, diced
1 cup	yellow onion, chopped (5.5 ounces)
1/2 cup	carrot, peeled and chopped (2.5 ounces)
1/2 cup	celery, chopped (2 ounces)
1 lb	button mushrooms, sliced
1/4 cup	red wine
3	cans low fat beef broth (14-ounces each)
1 ounce	dehydrated exotic mushrooms (chanterelles, porcinis or shitakes)
1 tbsp	fresh parsley, minced
1 tsp	fresh thyme leaves
1	bay leaf
2 tbsps	tomato paste
1/2 cup	heavy cream

Bring 1 can of beef broth to a boil in a small saucepan. Once it comes to a boil, add the dehydrated mushrooms and allow them to reconstitute for at least 30 minutes. Heat a large Dutch oven over medium high heat. Add the diced bacon and allow the fat to begin to render. Once it has rendered and the bacon begins to color, add the onion, carrot and celery. Sauté for 7-8 minutes, until the onion begins to brown. Stir in the red wine and allow it to reduce nearly completely. Add the button mushrooms and tomato paste, stirring constantly until the mushrooms begin to release their juices. Add the remaining cans of beef broth, the parsley, thyme and bay leaf. Turn the heat to medium low and simmer for 30-35 minutes, until the mushrooms and other vegetables are very tender. Drain the dehydrated mushrooms, saving the broth to add to the soup. Remove the bay leaf, then with either a stand blender or an immersion blender, purée the soup until smooth. Stir in the heavy cream and add the roughly chopped reconstituted mushrooms. Allow to simmer 10-15 minutes more before serving.

Lunch

Eucalorics

Corn and Crab Pasta Salad

6 Portions • 300 Calories, 9 grams of Fat

1 lb	cooked lump crabmeat
8 ounces	penne pasta
10 ounces	whole kernel frozen corn
3/4 cup	celery, diced (3 ounces)
3/4 cup	red bell pepper, diced (3 ounces)
1/3 cup	scallions, sliced thin
1 cup	reduced fat mayonnaise
1 cup	light sour cream
1 tbsp	Old Bay seasoning
1/2 tsp	kosher salt
	pinch black pepper

Microwave corn for 5 minutes, to thaw and cook slightly. Set aside and allow to cool. Bring a large pot of salted water to a boil over high heat. Cook penne according to the package directions, then rinse and drain. Pick over the crab to check for any pieces of shell. Combine crab with corn, celery, red bell pepper and scallions. In a small bowl combine mayonnaise, sour cream, Old Bay seasoning, salt and pepper. Combine with crab. Salad may be chilled several hours, or served immediately.

Lunch

Italian Ham and Mozzarella Melt

1 Portion • 355 Calories, 14.5 grams of Fat

1	2-ounce Italian roll
2 ounces	lean deli ham
1 ounce	part-skim mozzarella
1	Roma tomato
1/2 tbsp	unsalted butter
	pinch granulated garlic powder
	pinch dried basil leaf

Preheat the broiler. Spread the roll with butter and sprinkle with garlic powder. Top one half with ham, then cheese, then sliced tomato. Sprinkle with basil. Place both halves of the sandwich under the broiler and toast until the cheese is melted and the bread begins to brown.

Lunch

Eucalorics

Tarragon Chicken Salad

6 Portions • 215 Calories, 8 grams of Fat

1 recipe	Poached Chicken for Salad (pg. 149)
1	Granny Smith apple, peeled and diced (5 ounces)
1 ounce	walnut pieces, toasted
3/4 cup	celery, diced (3 ounces)
2 tbsps	scallions, sliced thin
1/2 cup	reduced fat mayonnaise
1/4 cup	light sour cream
2 tsps	fresh tarragon, minced
3/4 tsp	kosher salt
	pinch black pepper

Combine chicken, apple, walnuts, celery and scallions in a large bowl. Stir together mayonnaise, sour cream, tarragon, salt and pepper. Toss the tarragon dressing with the chicken mixture. Salad may be chilled several hours or served immediately.

Lunch

Marinated Asparagus

6 Portions • 60 Calories, 5 grams of Fat

24 ounces	asparagus
2 tbsps	olive oil
1 tbsp	tarragon vinegar*
	kosher salt
	ground black pepper

*A good-quality white wine vinegar may be substituted for the tarragon vinegar.

Bring a large pot of water to a boil. Wash asparagus and trim the woody ends (last 2-3 inches) from the spears. Boil for 2 minutes, drain and rinse under cold water. Pat dry.

Whisk together the oil and vinegar. Toss with the asparagus and season with salt and pepper. Refrigerate for at least 15 minutes before serving.

Lunch

Eucalorics

Soft Bean Burrito

1 Portion • 465 Calories, 14 grams of Fat

2	1-ounce flour tortillas
1/2 cup	canned fat free refried beans
1/4 cup	yellow onion, chopped (1.5 ounces)
1 ounce	Mexican-blend cheese, shredded
1/4 cup	hot sauce

Preheat the oven to 350 degrees. In a bowl combine the beans, onion, half the cheese and 2 tbsps of hot sauce. Divide the bean mixture between the two tortillas. Then top each tortilla with cheese and remaining 2 tbsps of hot sauce. Wrap up the burritos and bake for 15 minutes, until the burritos are heated through and the cheese is melted.

Cream of Chicken Corn Soup

6 Portions • 175 Calories, 6 grams of Fat

1 tbsp	unsalted butter
1/2 cup	yellow onion, chopped (2.5 ounces)
1/2 cup	celery, chopped (2 ounces)
8 ounces	whole kernel frozen corn
12 ounces	boneless skinless chicken breast
2 cups	fat free chicken broth
2 cups	whole milk
1/3 cup	all-purpose flour
1 tbsp	freeze-dried chives
1/2 tsp	kosher salt
1/8 tsp	black pepper

Place chicken in a large saucepan and cover with cold water. Bring to a boil over high heat, then turn to low and simmer the chicken for 15-20 minutes, until cooked through. Cut into bite-sized pieces.

Heat the butter in a large dutch oven over medium low heat. Add the onion and celery and sauté until the onion begins to soften, about five minutes. Add the corn and chicken broth and allow to simmer for 15 minutes, until the corn is cooked and the celery is tender. Whisk together the flour and milk. Add to the pot along with the chicken, chives, salt and pepper. Bring the soup to a gentle boil and thicken. Turn to low and simmer at least 15 minutes before serving.

Eucalorics

Cornbread

6 Portions • 155 Calories, 5 grams of Fat

1/2 cup	all-purpose flour (2.5 ounces)
1/2 cup	yellow cornmeal (2.5 ounces)
2 tbsps	granulated sugar
1 tsp	baking powder
1/2 tsp	kosher salt
3/4 cup	skim milk
1	large egg, divided
2 tbsps	unsalted butter, melted

Whisk together the flour, cornmeal, sugar, baking powder and salt. Combine the milk and the egg yolk and stir into the cornmeal mixture. Beat the egg white to soft peaks by hand or with a mixer. Fold first the egg white into the cornmeal, then the melted butter. Coat an 8x8 inch ovenproof pan with cooking spray. Place the batter in the pan in an even layer. Place in the oven for 35-40 minutes, until the cornbread is cooked through.

Lunch

Sloppy Joes

6 Portions • 230 Calories, 4 grams of fat

1 lb	96% extra lean ground beef
2 tbsps	dehydrated onion flakes
3/4 cup	ketchup
1 tbsp	brown sugar (packed)
1 tbsp	yellow mustard
1 tbsp	distilled white vinegar
6	hamburger buns (1.5 ounces each)

In a large skillet, brown the ground beef stirring frequently to break up beef. When the beef is cooked through, add the onion, ketchup, mustard, vinegar and brown sugar. Allow to simmer for 10-15 minutes, until the sauce has thickened and heated through. Divide the mixture between the 6 hamburger buns.

Lunch

Eucalorics

Mandarin Chicken Salad

1 Portion • 265 Calories, 5 grams of Fat

2 cups	romaine lettuce
1	4-ounce boneless, skinless chicken breast filet
2 tbsps	scallions, sliced thin
1 tbsp	sliced almonds
1/2 cup	mandarin orange segments
1	Recipe Asian Vinaigrette (below)

Grill or broil the chicken breast until cooked through, 6-8 minutes per side. Slice chicken into thin strips, then toss with lettuce, almonds and mandarin oranges. Top with Asian Vinaigrette.

Asian Vinaigrette

1 tbsp	seasoned rice vinegar
2 tsps	canola oil
1 tsp	toasted sesame oil
1 tbsp	fresh minced cilantro
1 tbsp	fresh minced mint
	pinch kosher salt

In a bowl whisk together vinegar and oils. Add cilantro, mint and salt. Allow to rest for at least 15 minutes before using.

1 Portion • 130 Calories, 14 grams of Fat

Open-Faced Chicken Quesadillas

2 portions • 445 Calories, 17.5 grams of Fat

2	1-ounce flour tortillas
1	4-ounce boneless, skinless chicken breast filet
1/2 cup	yellow onion, chopped (3 ounces)
2 tbsps	canned mild green chilies
1 tsp	canola oil
1 ounce	shredded Mexican-blend cheese
1 serving	Fresh Tomato Salsa (below)

Preheat the broiler. Heat the oil in a medium-size nonstick skillet. Finely dice the raw chicken. Sauté the chicken with the onion and green chilies until cooked through, 10-12 minutes. Place the tortillas on a cookie sheet and top each with half of the chicken mixture, then top each tortilla with 2 tbsps of cheese. Broil for 5-7 minutes, until the cheese is melted and the tortillas are crisp around the edges. Top with fresh tomato salsa.

Fresh Tomato Salsa

1	Roma tomato, seeded and diced
1 tbsp	red onion, finely chopped
1 tsp	pickled jalapeno pepper, minced
1 tsp	fresh cilantro, minced
1 tsp	fresh lime juice
	pinch kosher salt

Combine all ingredients in a bowl and allow to rest at least 15 minutes before serving.

1 Portion • 35 Calories, 0 grams of Fat

Lunch

Eucalorics

Tuna Salad Sandwiches

6 Portions • 115 Calories, 4 grams of Fat

2	cans solid white albacore tuna in spring water (6-ounce)
1/4 cup	yellow onion, chopped (2 ounces)
1/2 cup	celery, chopped (2 ounces)
1	large egg, hardboiled and grated
1/2 cup	reduced fat mayonnaise
2 tbsps	sweet pickle relish

Flake tuna into small pieces before adding the onion, celery, egg, mayonnaise and pickle relish. Mix until salad is well-combined. Chill or serve immediately.

Lunch

Cajun Chicken Salad

6 Portions • 225 Calories, 8 grams of Fat

1 recipe	Poached Chicken for Salad (pg. 149)
1 ounce	Andouille sausage
3/4 cup	celery, diced (3 ounces)
1/4 cup	green bell pepper, diced (1 ounce)
1/4 cup	red onion, diced (1.5 ounces)
1/4 cup	scallions, sliced
1 clove	garlic, minced
1/3 cup	reduced fat mayonnaise
1/2 cup	light sour cream
1 tbsp	Cajun Seasoning (pg. 195)

Finely dice the andouille sausage. Place in a medium nonstick skillet and heat over medium heat. When the fat begins to render, add the celery, onion and bell pepper. Sauté until the vegetables have softened, 5-7 minutes. Remove from the heat and allow to cool. Combine the chicken, sautéed vegetables and sausage. In a small bowl mix together the garlic, mayonnaise, sour cream, scallions and Cajun seasoning. Toss the chicken mixture with the Cajun dressing. Salad may be chilled several hours, or served immediately.

Lunch

Minestrone Soup

6 portions • 230 calories, 2.5 grams of fat

1/2 tbsp	olive oil
2 ounces	country ham, diced
1/2 cup	yellow onion, chopped (2.5 ounces)
1 clove	garlic, minced
1/4 cup	carrot, peeled and chopped (1 ounce)
1/4 cup	celery, chopped (1 ounce)
2	cans fat free chicken broth (14-ounce)
1	can petite diced tomatoes (28 ounces)
10 ounces	shredded green cabbage
1/4 cup	frozen cut green beans (2 ounces)
1/4 cup	frozen green peas (1 ounce)
1	can Navy beans, rinsed and drained (16-ounce)
1 tbsp	dried basil
1/2 tsp	dried oregano
4 ounces	elbow macaroni

Heat the olive oil in a large Dutch oven over medium high heat. Add the diced ham, onion, garlic, carrot and celery. Sauté for 7-8 minutes, until the onion begins to brown. Stir in the chicken broth, tomatoes, cabbage, green beans, peas, navy beans, basil and oregano. Bring to a boil, then stir in the macaroni. Turn the soup down to low and simmer for 30-40 minutes, until the pasta is cooked and the green beans and peas are tender.

Sun Dried Tomato and Parmesan Focaccia

6 portions • 215 Calories, 6 grams of Fat

12 ounces	plain focaccia bread
2 tbsps	Sun dried tomatoes, packed in oil
4 ounces	Parmesan cheese, finely grated

Preheat oven to 400 degrees, split focaccia in half. Mince sun dried tomatoes and mix with cheese. Place cheese on bottom half of focaccia. Place top over cheese and wrap in foil. Bake for 10-15 minutes until the cheese has melted. Unwrap and cut into six wedges.

Chicken Cacciatore with Buttered Macaroni

6 portions • 405 Calories, 8.5 grams of Fat

6	4-ounce boneless, skinless chicken breast filets
2 tbsps	olive oil
3 cups	yellow onion, sliced thin (12 ounces)
2	large bell peppers, sliced thin (11 ounces)
8 ounces	button mushrooms, sliced
6 cloves	garlic, minced
1	can diced tomatoes in sauce (14.5-ounce)
1	can crushed tomatoes (15-ounce)
1	can tomato paste (6-ounce)
1 1/2 tbsps	dried basil leaf
1/2 tsp	dried oregano
1/2 tsp	kosher salt
1/4 tsp	crushed red pepper flakes
8 ounces	macaroni
1/2 tbsp	unsalted butter

Heat oil over medium high heat in a large Dutch oven. Pat the chicken breasts dry, then season with salt and pepper. Brown the chicken in the oil, 4-5 minutes per side. Place the chicken on a plate.

Add the onions, bell peppers, mushrooms and garlic to the pan. Sauté for 5 minutes, until the onions and bell peppers begin to soften and the mushrooms release their liquid. Stir in the tomato products, basil, oregano, salt and red pepper flakes. Return the chicken to the pan and allow to simmer 25-30 minutes.

While the cacciatore is simmering, bring a large pot of salted water to a boil. Cook the macaroni according to the package directions. Drain well and toss with butter.

Mushroom Smothered Chicken

6 Portions • 190 Calories, 6.5 grams of Fat

6	4-ounce boneless skinless chicken breasts
1 tbsp	canola oil
1 tbsp	unsalted butter
1/2 cup	yellow onion, chopped (2.5 ounces)
1 clove	garlic, minced
1/2 cup	red wine
1 lb	pound button mushrooms, sliced
1/2 cup	fat free chicken broth
1 tsp	red wine vinegar
2 tbsps	all-purpose flour
	kosher salt
	black pepper

Pat the chicken breasts dry, then season with salt and pepper. Heat the oil and butter in a large skillet over medium high heat. Brown the chicken in the oil and butter mixture, 4-5 minutes per side. Put the chicken on a plate.

Add the onions and garlic to the skillet and cook, stirring frequently, until the garlic begins to brown and the onions become translucent. Deglaze the pan with wine and allow it to reduce until only a tablespoon remains. Add the mushrooms, stirring constantly until the mushrooms release their juice.

In a medium bowl, whisk together the flour, chicken broth and red wine vinegar. Add the mixture to the skillet and bring to a boil, stirring constantly until the sauce is thickened and smooth. Return the chicken to the skillet, turn the heat to low and cover the skillet. Allow the chicken to simmer in the sauce for 10-15 minutes, until the chicken is cooked through.

Main Courses

Chipotle Chicken

6 Portions • 155 Calories, 2 grams of Fat

6	4-ounce boneless, skinless chicken breast filets
1/3 cup	ketchup
2 tbsps	light corn syrup
1 tbsp	granulated sugar
1 tsp	brown sugar (packed)
1 tsp	dehydrated onion flakes
1/2 tsp	dehydrated minced garlic
1/4 tsp	ground cumin seed
1 tsp	chipotle peppers in adobo sauce
1/3 cup	tomato juice

In a small saucepan combine the ketchup, corn syrup, granulated sugar, brown sugar, onion, garlic, cumin, chipotle peppers and tomato juice. Allow the sauce to come to a boil over medium heat, stirring occasionally. Remove from the stove and allow to cool slightly. Remove and reserve 1/3 cup of chipotle sauce for the Chipotle Ranch Dressing, pg. 232. Use remaining sauce to baste the chicken while broiling or grilling, 6-8 minutes per side.

Honey Mustard Chicken

6 Portions • 235 Calories, 6 grams of Fat

6	4-ounce boneless, skinless chicken breast filets
1 tbsp	canola oil
1 tbsp	unsalted butter
1/3 cup	honey
2 tbsps	Dijon mustard
2 tbsps	all-purpose flour
1/2 cup	fat free chicken broth
	kosher salt
	black pepper

Pat the chicken breasts dry, then season with salt and pepper. Heat the oil and butter in a large skillet over medium high heat. Brown the chicken in the oil and butter mixture, 4-5 minutes per side. Put the chicken on a plate.

In a medium bowl, whisk together the honey, mustard, flour and broth. Add to the skillet and bring to a boil. Once the sauce thickens, return the chicken to the pan and cover it. Allow the chicken to simmer in the sauce over low heat for 10-15 minutes, until the chicken is cooked through.

Main Courses

Eucalorics

Barbecue Chicken

6 Portions • 185 Calories, 2 grams of Fat

6	4-ounce boneless skinless chicken breast filets
1 cup	homemade or store-bought barbecue sauce

Preheat grill or broiler. Toss the chicken with 1/2 cup of sauce. Grill or broil until cooked through, 6-8 minutes per side, basting the chicken with the remaining sauce.

Onion and Rosemary Chicken

6 Portions • 165 Calories, 5.5 grams of Fat

6	4-ounce boneless, skinless chicken breast filets
1 1/2 tbsps	olive oil
1 cup	yellow onion, sliced thin (4 ounces)
3 cloves	garlic, minced
1 tsp	lemon zest
1 tbsp	fresh rosemary
1/2 tsp	kosher salt
1/8 tsp	black pepper

Preheat the oven to 350 degrees. In a bowl, combine the oil, onion, garlic, lemon zest, rosemary, salt and pepper. Place the chicken breasts flat in a large foil-lined baking pan. Top with onion mixture. Place in oven and bake until chicken is cooked through and the onions are tender, 25-30 minutes.

Teriyaki Chicken

6 Portions • 220 Calories, 2 grams of Fat

6	4-ounce boneless, skinless chicken breast filets
1 cup	low sodium soy sauce
1/4 cup	Japanese rice wine (Mirin)
2 cloves	garlic, minced
1 tsp	fresh ginger, minced
4 tbsps	packed brown sugar
2 tbsps	granulated sugar
3 tbsps	cornstarch

In a medium bowl, combine the soy sauce, rice wine, garlic, ginger and sugars. Add the chicken and marinate for at least 1 hour and up to overnight. Preheat grill or broiler. Grill or broil the chicken until cooked through, 6-8 minutes per side, reserving the teriyaki marinade. While the chicken is cooking, whisk the cornstarch into the teriyaki sauce, then place it in a small saucepan and bring it to a boil over medium high heat. Serve the sauce as an accompaniment to the cooked chicken.

Main Courses

Chicken and Mushroom Risotto

6 Portions • 360 Calories, 11 grams of Fat

1 1/2 lbs	boneless skinless chicken breast
1 cup	yellow onion, chopped (5.5 ounces)
2 cloves	garlic, minced
1 1/2 tbsps	olive oil
1 cup	Arborio rice (6 ounces)
1 pound	button mushrooms, sliced
1 cup	white wine
3 cups	fat free chicken broth
2 ounces	Parmesan cheese, finely grated
2 ounces	Gruyere cheese, finely grated

Place chicken in a large saucepan and cover with cold water. Bring to a boil over high heat, then turn to low and simmer the chicken for 15-20 minutes, until cooked through. Cut into bite-sized pieces.

Heat the oil in a large Dutch oven over medium high heat. Add the onions and garlic and sauté until the onions begin to soften and the garlic begins to color. Stir in the rice and cook for a 3-5 minutes, until it too begins to color. Then, turning the heat to medium low, add the white wine. Stirring frequently, allow the wine to come to a boil and reduce almost completely.

While the wine is reducing, bring the chicken broth to a boil in a small saucepan. Once the wine is evaporated, add 1 cup of broth to the rice. Stir frequently and allow it to simmer and be completely absorbed. Add the second cup of broth and the mushrooms and allow it to simmer until that broth is absorbed. Add the chicken with the final cup of broth. When nearly all the broth is absorbed, add the Parmesan and Gruyere cheeses, stirring until the cheese is melted and distributed throughout the risotto.

Tamale Pie with Cornbread Crust

6 Portions • 390 Calories, 10 grams of Fat

Chili Beef and Corn Filling

1 1/2 lbs	96% extra lean ground beef
1 1/2 cups	yellow onion, chopped (8 ounces)
10 ounces	frozen whole kernel corn
2 cloves	garlic, minced
3/4 tsp	kosher salt
1 1/2 tbsps	chili powder
1 1/2 tsps	ground cumin seed
1	can tomato sauce (28-ounce)
1	can petite diced tomatoes, drained (15-ounce)

Cornmeal Batter Crust

1/2 cup	all-purpose flour (2.5 ounces)
1/2 cup	yellow cornmeal (2.5 ounces)
1 tsp	baking powder
1/2 tsp	iodized salt
1/2 tsp	chili powder
1/4 tsp	ground cumin seed
1	large egg, separated
3/4 cup	skim milk
2 tbsps	unsalted butter, melted

Preheat the oven to 400 degrees. In a large Dutch oven, brown the ground beef with the onion and garlic, stirring to break up beef. When the meat is cooked, stir in the corn, chili powder, cumin, salt, crushed tomatoes, tomato sauce and drained diced tomatoes. Allow to simmer 15-20 minutes.

While the chili beef and corn filling is simmering, prepare the cornbread crust. In a large bowl, whisk together the flour, cornmeal, salt, chili powder and cumin seed. In a small bowl beat together the egg yolk and milk. In a stand mixer with the whip attachment, beat the egg white until soft peaks form. Stir the milk and egg yolk into the cornmeal mixture. Fold in the egg white and finally the melted butter.

Place the chili beef and corn filling in the bottom of a 8x8 inch baking dish. Cover with the cornmeal batter. Bake for 25-30 minutes, until the crust is set and golden brown.

Main Courses

Meatloaf

6 Portions • 185 Calories, 5 grams of Fat

1 1/2 lbs	96% extra lean ground beef
1/2 cup	old-fashioned rolled oats (1.5 ounces)
1/2 cup	skim milk
1/4 cup	yellow onion, chopped (1.5 ounces)
1/4 cup	celery, diced (1 ounce)
1	large egg
1 tsp	kosher salt
1/2 tsp	black pepper
1/2 tsp	granulated garlic powder
1/2 tsp	dry mustard
1 tbsp	Worcestershire Sauce

Preheat the oven to 350 degrees. Stir together the milk and egg, then add the oats. Allow the mixture to stand for 5 minutes. Stir in the onion, celery, salt, pepper, garlic, mustard and Worcestershire sauce. Combine thoroughly with the ground beef. Pack the meatloaf tightly into a large, 5x9 inch, loaf pan. Bake uncovered for 50-55 minutes, until the meatloaf reaches an internal temperature of 165 degrees.

Main Courses

Chili Mac

6 Portions • 400 Calories, 10 grams of Fat

1 lb	96% extra lean ground beef
1 cup	yellow onion, chopped (5.5 ounces)
1	large green bell pepper, chopped (5.5 ounce)
1 clove	garlic, crushed
1/2 tsp	kosher salt
1 1/2 tbsps	chili powder
1	can crushed tomatoes (28-ounce)
1	can tomato sauce (8-ounce)
1	can diced tomatoes, drained (15-ounce)
9 ounces	macaroni
4 ounces	cheddar cheese, finely shredded

Preheat the oven to 350 degrees. In a large Dutch oven, brown the ground beef with the onion, green pepper and garlic, stirring frequently to break up beef. When the beef is cooked through, add chili powder, salt, crushed tomatoes, tomato sauce and diced tomatoes. Allow to simmer 15-20 minutes.

While the chili mixture is simmering, bring a large pot of salted water to a boil over high heat. Cook macaroni according to the package directions. Drain well, then toss the macaroni with the chili sauce. Place in a 8x8 inch ovenproof baking dish and top with the cheddar cheese. Bake for 10-15 minutes, until the cheese is melted and the chili mac is bubbling around the edges.

Ground Beef Stroganoff with Buttered Egg Noodles

6 Portions • 335 Calories, 8 grams of Fat

1 lb	96% extra lean ground beef
1	packet onion soup mix (1-ounce)
8 ounces	button mushrooms, sliced
1	can cream of mushroom soup (10.75-ounce)
2 cups	low fat beef broth
9 ounces	wide egg noodles
1 tbsp	unsalted butter

In a large Dutch oven, brown the ground beef, stirring to break up. When the meat is cooked, stir in the mushrooms, onion soup mix, cream of mushroom soup and low fat beef broth. Allow the stroganoff to simmer 15-20 minutes.

While the stroganoff simmers, bring a large pot of salted water to a boil. Cook the egg noodles according to the package directions. Drain well and toss with butter. Divide the noodles into six servings and top each portion with the stroganoff.

Main Courses

Chili Stuffed Peppers

6 Portions • 210 Calories, 7 grams of Fat

1 lb	96% extra lean ground beef
1/3 cup	yellow cornmeal (1.5 ounces)
1/3 cup	tomato juice
1/4 cup	yellow onion, chopped (1.5 ounces)
1	large egg
1/2 tsp	chili powder
1/4 tsp	ground cumin seed
1/4 tsp	kosher salt
3	large green bell peppers (5.5 ounce)
1	can tomato sauce (16-ounce)
1 tsp	chili powder
1/2 tsp	ground cumin seed
2 ounces	shredded cheddar cheese

Preheat oven to 350 degrees. Bring a large pot of water to a boil over high heat. Halve bell peppers lengthwise and remove the veins and seeds. Boil the peppers for 5 minutes, then drain them. Place the peppers cut side up in a 9x13 inch ovenproof baking dish.

In a large bowl combine the ground beef, cornmeal, tomato juice, onion, egg, chili powder, cumin and salt. Divide the mixture between the six pepper halves, packing the filling into their cavities. Bake for 20 minutes. While the peppers are baking, combine the tomato sauce, chili powder and cumin in a small saucepan. Bring to a boil, then simmer for 15 minutes. After the peppers have baked for 20 minutes, top them with the chili sauce and cheese. Bake for 10 more minutes, until the cheese is melted and the peppers are cooked through.

Spaghetti with Meat Sauce

6 Portions • 405 Calories, 7 grams of Fat

1 lb	96% extra lean ground beef
1/2 cup	yellow onion, chopped (2.5 ounces)
3 cloves	garlic, minced
1	can crushed tomatoes (28-ounce)
1	can tomato sauce (8-ounce)
1 cup	low fat beef broth
1/2 tsp	dried basil leaf
1/4 tsp	dried thyme
1/4 tsp	dried oregano
1/4 tsp	kosher salt
	pinch black pepper
12 ounces	thin spaghetti
3 ounces	Parmesan cheese

In a large Dutch oven, brown the ground beef over medium high heat with the onion and garlic, stirring to break up. When meat is cooked, add the crushed tomatoes, tomato sauce, broth, basil, thyme, oregano, salt and pepper. Allow to simmer at least 15 minutes.

Bring a large pot of salted water to a boil. Cook the spaghetti according to package directions. Divide the pasta between six servings and top each with 1 cup of sauce and half an ounce of Parmesan cheese.

Black Pepper and Parmesan Shrimp Capellini

6 Portions • 370 Calories, 9 grams of Fat

1 tbsp	unsalted butter
1 tbsp	olive oil
3 cloves	garlic, minced
1/2 tsp	black pepper
1 tsp	anchovy paste
2 tbsps	all-purpose
1	bottle clam juice (8-ounce)
9 ounces	cooked, peeled shrimp
12 ounces	capellini (angel hair) pasta
2 ounces	Parmesan cheese, finely shredded
2	Roma tomatoes, seeded and chopped
1/4 cup	scallions, sliced thin

Bring a large pot of salted water to a boil. Place butter, oil, garlic and black pepper in a cold nonstick skillet. Over medium high heat, melt the butter and cook the garlic until slightly golden. Stir in the anchovy paste and cook for 1 minute. Add the flour and cook for 2-3 minutes. Add the clam juice and bring to a boil, stirring until it thickens. Cook the pasta according to the package directions. Add the shrimp to the sauce and toss until warm. Drain the pasta well. Add the pasta, Parmesan, tomatoes and scallions to the sauce and toss to coat.

Main Courses

Linguine with White Clam Sauce

6 Portions • 355 Calories, 9.5 grams of Fat

2 tbsps	olive oil
2 tbsps	unsalted butter
1 cup	yellow onion, chopped (5.5 ounces)
3 cloves	garlic, minced
1/8 tsp	diced red pepper flakes
3	cans chopped clams (6.5-ounce)
1	bottle clam juice (8-ounce)
3 tbsps	all-purpose flour
1/4 cup	fresh parsley, chopped
12 ounces	linguine

Bring a large pot of salted water to a boil. Heat the olive oil in a large nonstick skillet over medium high heat. Add the onion, garlic and red pepper flakes. Sauté until the onion becomes translucent and the garlic begins to lightly color. Stir in the flour, stirring constantly until the flour is lighty browned and thickened. Drain and reserve the juice from the canned clams. Add reserved juice and the bottled clam juice to the roux and allow the sauce to thicken and become smooth. Add the clams. Cook the linguine according to the package instructions. Drain and toss with butter before tossing with the clam sauce and parsley.

Andouille and Crawfish Trinity

6 Portions • 185 Calories, 8.5 grams of Fat

4 ounces	Andouille sausage
1 lb	cooked crawfish tailmeat*
2 cloves	garlic, minced
1/2 cup	yellow onion, chopped (2.5 ounces)
1/2 cup	celery, sliced (2 ounces)
1/2 cup	bell pepper, chopped (2.5 ounces)
3 cups	fat free chicken broth
1/4 cup	all-purpose flour
2 tsps	dried basil leaf
1 tsp	dried thyme
1/2 tsp	sweet paprika
1/2 tsp	kosher salt
	black pepper

*shrimp may be substituted for the crawfish

Quarter the Andouille sausage lengthwise, then cut into quarter-inch slices. Place in a large nonstick skillet. Brown the sausage over medium high heat. After the fat has begun to render, 2-3 minutes, add the onion, celery, bell pepper and garlic. Cook until the vegetable trinity begins to soften and the garlic begins to brown. Stir in the basil, thyme, paprika, salt and black pepper. Whisk together the flour and chicken broth. Add the broth to the pan. Allow the broth to come to a boil and thicken. When the sauce is thick and smooth, stir in the crawfish to heat through. Serve over the Scallion and Parsley Pilaf (Pg. 201).

Garlic and Pepper Pork Loin

6 Portions • 170 Calories, 6.5 grams of Fat

1	2-pound center-cut pork loin
2 cloves	garlic
1 tsp	black pepper
2 tsps	kosher salt
1/2 tbsp	olive oil

Preheat oven to 325 degrees. Peel the garlic and use a mortar and pestle to mash the garlic, pepper, salt and oil into a paste. Pat the pork loin dry and rub with the garlic and pepper paste. Allow the meat to marinate for at least 15 minutes and up to overnight. Place the pork loin in the oven and roast for 50-55 minutes, until the loin reaches an internal temperature of 145 degrees. Remove from the oven, cover with foil and allow the meat to rest for at least 15 minutes before slicing and serving.

Barbecue Rub Pork Loin

6 Portions • 175 Calories, 5.5 grams of Fat

1	2-pound center-cut pork loin
1 tbsp	sweet paprika
2 tsps	granulated sugar
1 tsp	packed brown sugar
1 tsp	granulated onion powder
1/2 tsp	granulated garlic powder
1 tsp	kosher salt
1/2 tsp	black pepper

Preheat oven to 325 degrees. Combine dry ingredients. Pat the pork loin dry and rub with the barbecue spice. Place the pork loin in the oven and roast for 50-55 minutes, until the loin reaches an internal temperature of 145 degrees. Remove it from the oven, cover with foil and allow the meat to rest for at least 15 minutes before slicing and serving.

Roasted Pork Loin with Mushroom Stuffing

6 Portions • 320 Calories, 9.5 grams of Fat

1	2 pound center-cut pork loin
	kosher salt
	ground black pepper

Preheat oven to 325 degrees. Pat pork loin dry and rub and season with salt and pepper. Place in the center of a 9x13 inch ovenproof baking dish. In a small saucepan heat the broth and butter, until the butter is melted. In a large bowl combine bread cubes, onion, celery, mushrooms, poultry seasoning, sage, thyme, salt and black pepper. Toss with the broth and butter mixture. Pack the stuffing around the pork. Place the dish in the oven and roast the pork and stuffing until the loin reaches an internal temperature of 145 degrees, 50-55 minutes. Remove from the oven, cover with foil and allow the meat to rest for at least 15 minutes before slicing and serving.

Mushroom Stuffing

6 ounces	dry unseasoned bread cubes
1/2 cup	yellow onion, chopped (2.5 ounces)
1/2 cup	celery, chopped (2 ounces)
8 ounces	button mushrooms, sliced
1/2 tsp	poultry seasoning
1/2 tsp	rubbed sage
1/2 tsp	dried thyme
1/2 tsp	kosher salt
1/4 tsp	black pepper
1 1/2 cups	vegetable broth
1 tbsp	unsalted butter

Italian Seasoned Pork Loin

6 Portions • 165 Calories, 5.5 grams of Fat

2 lbs	center-cut pork loin
1 tsp	kosher salt
1 tsp	dried parsley flakes
1/2 tsp	dried basil leaf
1/2 tsp	granulated garlic powder
1/4 tsp	lemon pepper
1/8 tsp	crushed red pepper
1/8 tsp	dried oregano
	pinch dried rosemary

Preheat oven to 325 degrees. In a small bowl combine salt, parley, basil, garlic, lemon pepper, crushed red pepper, oregano and rosemary. Pat pork loin dry and rub with Italian herb seasoning. Allow the pork to marinate for 15 minutes to overnight. Roast in the oven for 50-55 minutes, until the loin reaches an internal temperature of 145 degrees. Remove from the oven, cover with foil and allow the meat to rest for at least 15 minutes before slicing and serving.

Main Courses

Rosemary and Thyme Roasted Pork

6 Portions • 165 Calories, 5.5 grams of Fat

2 lbs	center-cut pork loin
1 tbsp	fresh rosemary
1 tbsp	fresh thyme
1 clove	garlic, minced
1 tsp	lemon zest
1/2 tsp	kosher salt
	pinch ground black pepper

Preheat oven to 325 degrees. Mince together the garlic, lemon zest, rosemary and thyme. Pat pork loin dry, season with salt and pepper and rub with rosemary and thyme mixture. Allow the pork to marinate for 15 minutes to overnight. Roast in the oven for 50-55 minutes, until the loin reaches an internal temperature of 145 degrees. Remove from the oven, cover with foil and allow the meat to rest for at least 15 minutes before slicing and serving.

Main Courses

Cajun Pork Roast

6 Portions • 165 Calories, 5.5 grams of Fat

2 lbs	center-cut pork loin
2 tbsps	Cajun Seasoning

Preheat oven to 325 degrees. Pat pork loin dry and rub with the Cajun seasoning. Allow to marinate for at least 15 minutes and up to overnight. Roast in the oven for 50-55 minutes, until the loin reaches an internal temperature of 145 degrees. Remove from the oven, cover with foil and allow the meat to rest for at least 15 minutes before slicing and serving.

Cajun Seasoning

Yield: 1/2 cup

2 tbsps	paprika
2 tbsps	kosher salt
2 tsps	ground black pepper
1 tsp	ground white pepper
1 tsp	ground red (cayenne) pepper
1 1/2 tsps	granulated garlic powder
1 1/2 tsps	granulated onion powder
1 1/2 tsps	dried oregano
1 1/2 tsps	dried thyme

Combine all the herbs and spices and store in an airtight container.

1 teaspoon — 5 calories, 0 grams of Fat

Lemon Pollack

6 Portions • 165 Calories, 2 grams of Fat

6	6-ounce pollack filets
2	lemons
4 cups	water
1 tbsp	lemon pepper

Preheat the oven to 350 degrees. In a small saucepan bring water to a boil. Add the lemon pepper and allow to steep for 5 minutes. Arrange fish fillets in a single layer in a 9x13 inch baking dish. Cut each lemon in 6 slices. Season the fillets with salt and pepper and top with 2 lemon slices. Pour the lemon pepper broth over the fish. Place in the oven and bake for 30 minutes, until the fish begins to flake.

Spice Crusted Salmon Filets

6 Portions • 170 Calories, 6.5 grams of Fat

6	4-ounce salmon filets, skinned with bones removed
2 tbsps	whole cumin seed
1 tbsp	ground coriander seed
1 tbsp	whole fennel seed
1 tsp	kosher salt
1/2 tsp	black pepper

Preheat the oven to 350 degrees. Line a large baking sheet with foil. Place the salmon filets skin-side down. In a small bowl combine the cumin, coriander, fennel, salt and black pepper. Press 2 rounded teaspoons of the spice mixture onto each of the salmon filets. Bake for 15-18 minutes, until the fish begins to flake.

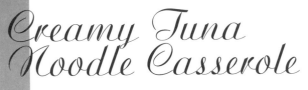

Creamy Tuna Noodle Casserole

6 Portions • 431 Calories, 12 grams of Fat

12 ounces	egg noodles
2	cans solid white albacore tuna in spring water (6-ounce)
2	cans cream of mushroom soup (10.75-ounce)
4 ounces	Light Velveeta® processed cheese
1 cup	pasta water, reserved

Bring a large pot of salted water to a boil and cook the noodles according to the package directions. Drain pasta, reserving 1 cup of the cooking liquid.

Combine the reserved liquid with the soup and cheese in a large sauce pan over medium heat. Once the cheese is melted, add the tuna, including juice, breaking it into small chunks. Add the noodles and continue to cook for 5 minutes more, until mixture is thoroughly combined and heated through.

Stuffed Flounder

6 Portions • 185 Calories, 6.5 grams of Fat

1 tbsp	unsalted butter
1/4 cup	scallions, sliced thin
1/4 cup	red onion, chopped (1.5 ounces)
3 ounces	imitation crabmeat
1/4 cup	sherry
1/4 cup	heavy cream
1/2 cup	cracker crumbs
6	4-ounce flounder filets
	kosher salt
	ground black pepper

Preheat the oven to 350 degrees. Melt the butter in a large skillet over medium high heat. Sauté the red onion and scallions for several minutes, until the onions begin to soften. Deglaze the pan with sherry and allow the liquid to reduce to a syrup. Add the cream and crab and reduce the cream by half. Stir in the cracker crumbs and continue to cook until the mixture holds together. Remove from the heat. Season the flounder filets with salt and pepper, then place 2 tablespoons of stuffing in the center of each fillet. With toothpicks secure the fillet around the stuffing. Place in an ovenproof pan and bake for 20 minutes, until the fish begins to flake.

Main Courses

Mustard and Cheese Cod Filets

6 Portions • 230 Calories, 7 grams of Fat

6	6-ounce cod filets
1	can cream of mushroom soup (10.75 ounce)
4 ounces	light Velveeta Cheese
1 tsp	dry mustard
	kosher salt
	black pepper

Preheat the oven to 350 degrees. In a small saucepan combine the cream of mushroom soup, cheese and dry mustard. Heat on medium until the cheese melts and the sauce is smooth. Place the cod filets in a 9x13 inch baking dish. Cover with the cheese sauce.

Place in the oven and bake for 20-25 minutes, until the cod just begins to flake.

Main Courses

Eucalorics

Scallion and Parsley Pilaf

6 Portions • 170 Calories, 2 grams of Fat

1 tbsp	unsalted butter
1 1/2 cups	basmati rice (9 ounces)
3 cups	water
1 tsp	kosher salt
1/8 tsp	black pepper
1/4 cup	fresh parsley, minced
1/4 cup	scallions, sliced thin

Melt the butter in a large nonstick skillet, over medium high heat. Add the rice to the pan and allow it to brown slightly, 4-5 minutes. Stir in the salt, pepper and water. Bring to a boil, cover and turn heat to low. When the liquid has been absorbed, 20-25 minutes, stir in the parsley and scallions.

Helpful Tips

Parsley will keep longer if stored in a glass of water in the refrigerator.

Orzo Pilaf

6 Portions • 165 Calories, 2.5 grams of Fat

1 tbsp	unsalted butter
1 cup	basmati rice (6 ounces)
1/2 cup	orzo pasta (4 ounces)
1 tsp	kosher salt
1/2 tsp	black pepper
3 cups	fat free chicken broth

Melt the butter in a medium saucepan. Add the orzo and basmati rice and cook over medium heat until golden brown, 5-7 minutes. Stir in the salt, pepper and chicken broth. Bring to a boil, cover and cook over low heat until all the liquid is absorbed, 20-25 minutes.

Cranberry Wild Rice

6 Portions • 185 Calories, 2 grams of Fat

1 tbsp	unsalted butter
3/4 cup	basmati rice (4.5 ounces)
1/3 cup	parboiled wild rice (2 ounces)
2 1/2 cups	vegetable stock
1 cup	yellow onion, chopped (5.5 ounces)
1 clove	garlic, minced
1 tsp	kosher salt
1/8 tsp	black pepper
1/4 cup	scallions, sliced thin
2 tbsps	fresh parsley, minced
3 ounces	sweetened dried cranberries

Melt the butter in a medium saucepan. Sauté the onion and garlic, until the onion becomes translucent and the garlic begins to color. Stir in the rice and wild rice and cook 1 minute. Add the vegetable broth, salt and pepper. Bring the broth to a boil, cover and cook over low heat until all the liquid is absorbed, 25-30 minutes. Remove from the heat and stir in the scallions, parsley and cranberries. Cover and allow to stand 5 minutes before serving.

Mexican Rice

6 Portions • 175 Calories, 1 gram of Fat

1 tsp	canola oil
1 1/2 cups	basmati rice (9 ounces)
1/4 cup	yellow onion, chopped (1.5 ounces)
1/4 cup	bell pepper, chopped (1.5 ounces)
1 tbsp	canned mild green chilies, chopped
2 cloves	garlic, minced
1 cup	tomato juice
2 cups	low fat beef broth
1 tsp	chili powder
1/4 tsp	ground cumin seed
1 1/2 tsps	kosher salt

Heat the oil over medium high heat in a medium saucepan. Add the onions, garlic and bell peppers and sauté for 5 minutes, until the onions become translucent. Stir in the rice, chilies, chili powder, cumin and salt. Cook for 1 minute. Add the tomato juice and beef broth and bring to a boil. Turn to low and cover the pan, allowing the rice to simmer 20-25 minutes, until all the liquid has absorbed.

Starches

Ham and Parmesan Orzo

6 Portions • 210 Calories, 5.5 grams of Fat

1 tbsp	unsalted butter
8 ounces	orzo pasta
2 ounces	Canadian bacon
2 ounces	grated Parmesan cheese
1 clove	garlic, minced
1 tsp	kosher salt
1/8 tsp	ground black pepper
1/8 tsp	lemon pepper
2 cups	water

Melt the butter in a large skillet over medium high heat. Add the garlic and bacon and sauté until the garlic begins to color lightly. Stir in the orzo and continue to stir until the pasta turns a golden brown. Stir in salt, black and lemon peppers. Add the water and bring to boil. Cover and turn the heat down to low. Cook for 25 minutes. Uncover the orzo and stir in the Parmesan cheese, cooking for 5 more minutes, stirring frequently until the cheese is melted and the remaining liquid is absorbed.

Red Beans and Rice

6 Portions • 205 Calories, 4 grams of Fat

2 ounces	Andouille sausage
1/2 cup	yellow onion, chopped (2.5 ounces)
1	clove garlic, minced
3/4 cup	basmati rice (4.5 ounces)
1	can diced tomatoes (14.5-ounce)
2 cups	tomato juice
1	can kidney beans (16-ounce)
1 tsp	Cajun seasoning (pg. 195)
1/4 tsp	kosher salt

Quarter the Andouille sausage lengthwise, then cut into 1/4 inch slices. Place in a large nonstick skillet. Brown the sausage over medium high heat. After the fat has begun to render, 2-3 minutes, add the onions and garlic. Cook until the onions become translucent and the garlic becomes fragrant. Stir in the rice, diced tomatoes, tomato juice, Cajun seasoning and salt. Bring the broth to a boil, cover and cook over low heat until the rice is tender and most of the liquid has absorbed, 20-25 minutes. Uncover, stir in the beans and cook 5 more minutes.

Starches

Orzo Primavera

6 Portions • 190 Calories, 5.5 grams of Fat

1 tbsp	butter
8 ounces	orzo pasta
1 cup	large red bell pepper, chopped (5.5 ounce)
1 cup	red onion, chopped (5.5 ounces)
1 cup	carrot, peeled and sliced thin (5 ounces)
3 cloves	fresh garlic, minced
1 tsp	kosher salt
1/2 tsp	basil leaf
1/8 tsp	dried oregano
1/8 tsp	crushed red pepper flakes
2 cups	fat free chicken broth

Melt the butter in a large skillet over medium high heat. Add the bell pepper, onions, carrots and garlic and sauté until the onions become translucent. Stir in the orzo and continue to stir until the pasta turns a golden brown. Stir in salt, basil, oregano and red pepper flakes and cook 1 more minute. Add the broth and bring to boil. Cover and turn the heat down to low. Cook for 20-25 minutes until the orzo is tender and the broth is completely absorbed.

Lemon Pepper Orzo

6 Portions • 175 Calories, 4.5 grams of Fat

2 tbsps	unsalted butter
8 ounces	orzo pasta
1 tsp	lemon pepper
1 tsp	kosher salt
2 cups	water

Melt the butter in a medium saucepan. Add the orzo and cook over medium heat until golden brown, 5-7 minutes. Stir in the salt, lemon pepper and water. Bring to a boil, cover and cook over low heat until all the liquid is absorbed, 20-25 minutes.

Starches

Golden Garlic Mashed Potatoes

6 Portions • 155 Calories, 4 grams of Fat

2 lbs	Yukon Gold Potatoes, peeled and chopped (6 cups)
6 cloves	garlic
1 1/2 tbsps	olive oil
1/2 cup	fat free chicken broth
1 tsp	kosher salt
1/4 tsp	ground black pepper

Preheat oven to 400 degrees. Peel the garlic cloves and place them in a small ovenproof container. Add oil and cover with foil. Bake the garlic for 40-45 minutes, until soft.

Cover potatoes with cold, salted water. Bring to a boil over high heat and cook until tender, 20-30 minutes. Drain well. Place in the bowl of a stand mixer. Add the garlic and olive oil, chicken broth, salt and pepper. Whip the potatoes smooth.

Buttermilk Mashed Potatoes

6 Portions • 145 Calories, 2 grams of Fat

2 lbs	russet or Idaho potatoes, peeled and chopped (6 cups)
1 tbsp	unsalted butter
1/2 cup	1% buttermilk
1 tsp	kosher salt
1/4 tsp	black pepper

Cover potatoes with cold, salted water. Bring to a boil over high heat and cook until tender, 20-30 minutes. Drain well. Place in the bowl of a stand mixer. Add butter, buttermilk, salt and pepper. Whip the potatoes smooth.

Starches

Helpful Tips

To keep potatoes from turning brown, cover them with water and the juice of one lemon or 2 tbsps white vinegar.

Eucalorics

Mustard Potato Salad

6 Portions • 160 Calories, 4.5 grams of Fat

1 1/2 lbs	red potatoes
1/2 cup	reduced fat mayonnaise
1 tbsp	yellow mustard
1/4 cup	onion, chopped (1.5 ounces)
1/4 cup	celery, diced (1 ounce)
2 tbsps	sweet pickle relish
2	large eggs, hard-boiled and grated
1/2 tsp	kosher salt
1/2 tsp	granulated sugar
1/8 tsp	black pepper

Cover potatoes with cold, salted water. Bring to a boil and cook until just tender, 20 25 minutes. Drain well. In a bowl combine mayonnaise, mustard, onion, celery, pickle relish, eggs, salt and pepper. When the potatoes are cool enough to handle, dice the potatoes into bite-sized chunks. Toss with dressing. Serve warm or chill and serve cold.

Cheddar and Chive Mashed Potatoes

6 Portions • 175 Calories, 4 grams of Fat

2 lbs	russet or Idaho potatoes, peeled and chopped (6 cups)
2 ounces	cheddar cheese, shredded (1/2 cup)
1 tbsp	freeze dried chives
1/4 cup	light sour cream
1/3 cup	skim milk
1 tsp	kosher salt
1/8 tsp	black pepper

Cover potatoes with cold, salted water. Bring to a boil over high heat and cook until tender, 20-30 minutes. Drain well. Place in the bowl of a stand mixer. Add the cheese, chives, sour cream, milk, salt and pepper. Whip the potatoes until smooth.

Starches

Parsley and Buttered New Potatoes

6 Portions • 155 Calories, 4 grams of Fat

2 lbs	new potatoes
2 tbsps	unsalted butter
1/4 cup	fresh parsley, minced
1 tsp	kosher salt
1/4 tsp	black pepper

Leave potatoes whole or halve depending on their size. Place in a large pot and cover with cold, salted water. Bring to a boil and cook until fork tender, 30-40 minutes, depending on the size of the potatoes. Drain well and toss with butter, parsley, salt and pepper.

Roasted Fingerling Potatoes with Fennel

6 Portions • 190 Calories, 5 grams of Fat

2 lbs	fingerling potatoes*
1 bulb	fresh fennel, sliced thin (8 ounces)
2 cups	red onion, sliced thin (8 ounces)
4 cloves	garlic, peeled and smashed
1 tsp	kosher salt
1/2 tsp	black pepper
2 tbsps	canola oil

*small red potatoes may be substituted if fingerlings are unavailable

Preheat oven to 400 degrees. Halve fingerling potatoes. Toss with half of oil, salt and pepper. Place in a 9x13 inch baking dish and roast for 30 minutes. Toss fennel, onion and garlic with remaining tablespoon of oil. Add to potatoes and roast for an additional 30 minutes, stirring once, after 15 minutes.

Starches

Couscous with Currants

6 Portions • 210 Calories, 2 grams of Fat

1 1/2 cups	couscous (9 ounces)
3 cups	vegetable broth
1 tbsp	unsalted butter
1/4 cup	scallions sliced thin
1 tbsp	fresh parsley, minced
2 ounces	currants
1/2 tsp	kosher salt
	pinch black pepper

In a large saucepan, bring the stock, butter, salt and pepper to a boil. Remove from the heat, add the couscous and cover for 5 minutes. After 5 minutes, remove the lid and fluff the couscous with a fork. Stir in the scallions, parsley and currants.

Mexican Corn and Black Beans

6 Portions • 165 Calories, 2 grams of Fat

1 tsp	canola oil
1 cup	yellow onions, chopped (5.5 ounces)
1 clove	garlic, minced
1	can mild green chilies (4-ounce)
1 tsp	ground cumin seed
1	can diced tomatoes, drained (14.5-ounce)
20 ounces	frozen whole kernel corn
1	can black beans, rinsed and drained (15-ounce)
1 tsp	kosher salt

Heat oil in a large nonstick skillet over medium high heat. Sauté onion and garlic until the onion becomes translucent and the garlic begins to lightly color. Stir in the remaining ingredients. Cover and turn the heat down to medium low and allow the mixture to cook 15-20 minutes. Uncover and cook for 5-10 additional minutes, until liquid evaporates.

Starches

Eucalorics

Barley Pilaf

6 Portions • 175 Calories, 3.5 grams of Fat

1 cup	pearled barley (7 ounces)
2 tbsps	unsalted butter
1 cup	yellow onion, chopped (5.5 ounces)
1 cup	celery, chopped (4 ounces)
2	cans fat free chicken broth (14-ounce)
1/3 cup	scallions, sliced thin
2 tbsps	fresh minced parsley
1 tsp	kosher salt
1/4 tsp	black pepper

Melt the butter in a large skillet over medium high heat. Add the onion and celery and sauté until the onions become translucent. Stir in the barley and continue to stir until it begins to color. Stir in salt, black pepper and chicken broth and bring to boil. Cover and turn the heat down to low. Cook for 30-35 minutes, until the barley is tender and the broth has been completely absorbed. Uncover the barley and stir in the scallions and parsley.

Starches

Vegetable Lo Mein

6 Portions • 200 Calories, 4 grams of Fat

8 ounces	fresh lo mein noodles
1 cup	yellow onion, chopped (5.5 ounces)
1 cup	celery, sliced thin (4 ounces)
1 cup	carrot, peeled and sliced thin (5 ounces)
4 ounces	button mushrooms, sliced
2 cloves	garlic, minced
1 tbsp	peanut oil
1/2 cup	fat free chicken broth
2 tbsps	low sodium soy sauce
1 tsp	toasted sesame oil
1 tbsp	cornstarch
1/4 tsp	crushed red pepper flakes
1/4 cup	scallions, sliced thin

Bring a large pot of water to a boil. Prepare the noodles according to the package directions. In a large skillet, heat the peanut oil until almost smoking. Add the onions, carrot, celery, mushrooms and garlic and sauté until they just begin to soften. In a small bowl combine the chicken broth, soy sauce, sesame oil, chili flakes and cornstarch. Add to the pan and bring to a boil and thicken. Add the drained noodles, stirring to evenly coat with sauce. Stir in the scallions before serving

Roasted Asparagus

6 Portions • 20 Calories, 0 grams of Fat

24 ounces	asparagus
	nonstick cooking spray
	kosher salt
	ground black pepper

Preheat the oven to 400 degrees. Wash asparagus and trim the woody ends (last 2-3 inches) from the spears and discard. Arrange asparagus in a single layer on foil lined baking sheets. Coat the asparagus evenly with cooking spray. Roast 5-7 minutes, depending on the thickness of the spears. Remove from the oven and season with salt and pepper.

Helpful Tips

Thinner stalks of asparagus tend to be more tender and better for roasting.

Country Green Beans

6 Portions • 80 Calories, 2 grams of Fat

1 1/2 lbs	frozen green beans
1 tsp	canola oil
1 cup	yellow onion, chopped (5.5 ounces)
4 ounces	Canadian bacon, diced
1/4 tsp	crushed red pepper flakes
1/2 tsp	kosher salt
1/8 tsp	black pepper

Heat oil in a large stockpot over medium high heat. Sauté onion and bacon until the onion begins to soften. Stir in the green beans and red pepper flakes. Cover, and allow the beans to stew over low heat, stirring occasionally. After 1 hour, uncover the beans, and cook for 15-20 minutes more, until the excess liquid evaporates. Season with salt and pepper before serving.

Helpful Tips

"Seasoning": Canadian bacon is a great substitute for traditional bacon to cut back on fat when cooking southern-style vegetables

Green Beans with Red Onion and Red Pepper

6 Portions • 70 Calories, 2 grams of Fat

1 1/2 lbs	green beans, washed and trimmed
1 1/2 cups	red onion, sliced thin (6 ounces)
1 tbsp	unsalted butter
1/2 tsp	kosher salt
1/8 tsp	crushed red pepper flakes

Bring a large pot of water to a boil. Cook the green beans for 5 minutes, until tender crisp. Drain well and rinse with cold water to stop the beans from cooking further. Melt the butter in a large nonstick skillet over medium high heat. Add the red onions, salt and red pepper flakes. Sauté for 5-7 minutes, until the onions become tender. Add the beans to the pan and cook for 1-2 minutes to re-warm the beans and evenly distribute the onions and red pepper flakes.

Green Beans with Carrots and Bell Peppers

6 Portions • 70 Calories, 2 grams of Fat

1 1/2 lbs	green beans, washed and trimmed
1 cup	carrot, peeled and sliced thin (5 ounces)
1	large red bell pepper, sliced thin (5.5 ounce)
1 tbsp	unsalted butter
1/2 tsp	kosher salt
1/8 tsp	black pepper

Bring a large pot of water to a boil. Cook the green beans for 5 minutes, until tender crisp. Drain well and rinse with cold water to stop the beans from cooking further. Melt the butter in a large nonstick skillet over medium high heat. Add the carrot and peppers. Sauté for 5-7 minutes, until the peppers and carrots are tender. Add the beans to the pan and cook for 1-2 minutes to re-warm the beans and evenly distribute the carrots and peppers. Season with salt and pepper.

Vegetables

Rainbow Carrot and Pepper Sauté

6 Portions • 60 Calories, 2 grams of Fat

1 tbsp	unsalted butter
1	large green bell pepper, stripped (5 ounce)
1	large red bell pepper, stripped (5 ounce)
1	large yellow bell pepper, stripped (5 ounce)
2 cups	carrots, peeled and shredded (10 ounces)
1 tsp	kosher salt
1/4 tsp	black pepper

Melt the butter in a large non-stick skillet over medium high heat. Add the pepper strips and carrots. Sauté for 5-7 minutes, until the peppers are tender and the carrot shreds become slightly limp. Toss with salt and pepper.

Glazed Carrots

6 Portions • 70 Calories, 2 grams of Fat

1 lb	baby carrots
1 tbsp	unsalted butter
2 tbsps	granulated sugar
1/2 tsp	kosher salt
	pinch black pepper

Bring a large pot of water to a boil. Boil the carrots for 10-12 minutes, until tender. Drain well. In a non-stick skillet, melt the butter over medium high heat. Stir in the sugar, dissolving it in the butter. Add the carrots to the pan and toss to coat. Season with salt and pepper.

Buttered Carrots

6 Portions • 60 Calories, 2 grams of Fat

1 lb	baby carrots
1	can fat free chicken broth (14-ounce)
1 tbsp	unsalted butter
	kosher salt
	black pepper

In a large skillet bring broth and butter to a boil. Add the carrots and continue to boil until the broth has evaporated, 15-20 minutes. The carrots should be tender and coated with the broth and butter reduction. Season to taste with salt and pepper.

Spicy Green Beans

6 Portions • 70 Calories, 2 grams of Fat

1 1/2 lbs	green beans, washed and trimmed
1 tbsp	butter
2 cloves	garlic, minced
1 tsp	kosher salt
1 tsp	granulated sugar
1 tsp	crushed red pepper flakes

Bring a large pot of water to a boil. Cook the green beans for 5 minutes, until tender crisp. Drain the beans well and rinse with cold water to stop them from cooking further. In the same pot, combine the oil, garlic, salt, sugar and crushed red pepper flakes. Heat the pan over medium heat until the garlic begins to color and the sugar and salt dissolve. Add the beans to the pot, tossing them with the garlic and pepper flakes, until they are well distributed and the beans are reheated.

Vegetables

Basic Tossed Salad

6 Portions • 40 Calories, 0.5 grams of Fat

12 ounces	romaine or other dark leafy lettuce
1 cup	shredded carrot
1	medium cucumber, peeled and chopped (7 ounce)
1	medium bell pepper, seeded and chopped (4 ounce)
1 cup	celery, diced (4 ounces)
1 cup	cherry tomatoes

Wash and dry lettuce before chopping into bite-sized pieces. Toss with remaining ingredients.

Helpful Tips

The darker the green, the more vitamins and minerals it contains.

Creamy Italian Dressing

12 – 2 tablespoon Portions • 30 Calories, 1.5 grams of Fat

1/3 cup	reduced fat mayonnaise
1/2 cup	light sour cream
1/2 cup	skim milk
1 tbsp	white wine vinegar
3/4 tsp	lemon pepper
1/4 tsp	granulated garlic powder
1/4 tsp	kosher salt
1/8 tsp	dried parsley flakes
1/8 tsp	dried basil leaf
1/8 tsp	granulated onion powder
1/8 tsp	black pepper
1 tsp	granulated sugar
	pinch dried oregano

Whisk together all the ingredients in a bowl. Refrigerate at least 15 minutes before serving. The dressing will keep up to 1 week in the refrigerator.

Eucalorics

Ranch Dressing

12 – 2 tablespoon Portions • 25 Calories, 1.5 grams of Fat

2 tbsps	**ranch dressing mix**
1/2 cup	**reduced fat mayonnaise**
7 ounces	**skim milk**

Whisk together dressing mix, mayonnaise and milk until smooth. Refrigerate for at least 20 minutes before using. Will keep 2-3 days in the refrigerator.

Green Goddess Dressing

12 – 2 tablespoon Portions • 35 Calories, 2 grams of Fat

1/3 cup	reduced fat mayonnaise
1/2 cup	light sour cream
1/2 cup	skim milk
2 tbsps	fresh parsley
1/4 cup	scallion, sliced thin
1 clove	garlic, minced
1 tsp	anchovy paste
1 tbsp	white wine vinegar
1/4 tsp	kosher salt
	black pepper

Place ingredients in the bowl of a food processor. Process until the dressing is smooth and has acquired a pale green cast from the finely minced parsley and scallions. Refrigerate for at least 15 minutes before serving. The dressing will keep 2-3 days in the refrigerator.

Thousand Island Dressing

12 – 2 tablespoon Portions • 45 Calories, 2.5 grams of Fat

1 cup	reduced fat mayonnaise
1/4 cup	ketchup
2 tbsps	sweet pickle, minced
2 tbsps	sweet pickle juice
1/2 tsp	dehydrated onion flakes
1/4 tsp	kosher salt
	black pepper

Combine mayonnaise, ketchup, pickle, onion, pickle, juice, salt and pepper in a bowl. Refrigerate for at least 15 minutes before using. Will keep in the refrigerator up to one month.

Chipotle Ranch Dressing

6 Portions • 50 Calories, 2 grams of Fat

1 tbsp	ranch dressing mix
1/3 cup	low fat mayonnaise
1/2 cup	skim milk
1/3 cup	reserved chipotle sauce (pg. 175)

Whisk together dressing mix, mayonnaise, milk and chipotle sauce until smooth. Refrigerate for at least 20 minutes before using. Will keep 2-3 days in the refrigerator.

Vegetables

Sautéed Spinach with Onion

6 Portions • 65 Calories, 1 gram of Fat

1 1/2 lbs	fresh baby spinach*
1 tsp	canola oil
1/2 cup	yellow onion, chopped (2.5 ounces)
1/4 tsp	crushed red pepper flakes
1/2 tsp	kosher salt
1/4 tsp	granulated sugar

*chopped, frozen spinach may be substituted. Thaw and squeeze the spinach to remove excess water before adding it to the Dutch oven.

If using fresh spinach, wash and spin dry, before chopping into 1-inch pieces. In a large Dutch oven, heat the oil over medium high heat. Sauté the onions until it becomes translucent, then stir in the red pepper, salt and sugar. Cook for 1 minute. Turn the heat to medium low and add the spinach, stirring occasionally until tender, 3-4 minutes.

Creamy Coleslaw

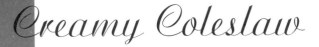

6 Portions • 75 Calories, 2.5 grams of Fat

1 1/2 lbs	prepared coleslaw mix
1/2 cup	reduced fat mayonnaise
2 1/2 tbsps	apple cider vinegar
1 1/2 tsps	granulated sugar
1/4 tsp	celery seed
1/2 tsp	kosher salt
1/8 tsp	black pepper

Combine mayonnaise, vinegar, sugar, celery seed, salt and black pepper. Toss with shredded slaw mix. (It will not look like enough dressing). Cover and refrigerate for at least 30 minutes before serving.

Garlic Zucchini

35 Calories, 2 grams of Fat

1 1/2 lbs	zucchini
1 tbsp	unsalted butter
3 cloves	garlic, minced
1/2 tsp	kosher salt
1/8 tsp	ground black pepper

Bring water to a boil in a 2-quart saucepan. Halve or quarter the zucchini lengthwise depending on the size. Slice zucchini into 3-inch sections. Boil zucchini for 3 minutes, drain well. In a nonstick skillet, melt the butter over medium high heat. Add the garlic, salt and pepper. Sauté the garlic until fragrant. Add the zucchini and toss to distribute the garlic butter.

Zucchini with Leeks

6 Portions • 40 Calories, 2 grams of Fat

1 1/2 lbs	zucchini
1	large leek
1 tbsp	unsalted butter
1/2 tsp	kosher salt
1/8 tsp	ground black pepper

Bring water to a boil in a 2-quart saucepan. Halve or quarter the zucchini lengthwise depending on the size. Slice zucchini into 3-inch sections. Boil zucchini for 3 minutes. Drain well.

Remove the stem end from the leek and cut in half. Wash well to remove any grit between the layers, then slice the white part of the leek into half moons. In a nonstick skillet, melt the butter over medium high heat. Add the leek and sauté until it is tender, 3-4 minutes. Add the zucchini to the skillet and toss with the onions. Season with salt and pepper.

Zucchini with Tomatoes and Cumin

6 Portions • 30 Calories, 1 gram of Fat

1 1/2 lbs	zucchini
1 tsp	canola oil
1 cup	tomato, chopped (6 ounces)
1 clove	garlic, minced
1 tsp	whole cumin seed
1 tsp	kosher salt
1/8 tsp	crushed red pepper flakes

Quarter the zucchini and cut into 1-inch chunks. Place oil, garlic, cumin seed and crushed red pepper in a cold non-stick skillet. Cook over medium high heat, until the cumin becomes fragrant and the garlic begins to color, 2-3 minutes. Add the tomatoes, zucchini and salt. Cover and turn the heat down to medium low. Allow to cook for 5-7 minutes, until the zucchini is tender. Uncover and cook over high heat until any liquid that had collected evaporates.

Vegetables

Tomatoes and Okra

6 Portions • 50 Calories, 1 gram of Fat

1 1/2 lbs	frozen okra
1 tsp	canola oil
1 cup	tomato, chopped (6 ounces)
1 clove	garlic, minced
1/2 tsp	kosher salt
1/8 tsp	ground black pepper

Bring a large pot of water to a boil. Cook the frozen okra for 10 minutes. Drain well. In the same pot, heat the oil over medium high. Add the garlic and sauté until it begins to color, 2-3 minutes. Add the tomatoes, okra, salt and pepper. Cook the tomatoes and okra, stirring frequently, until the tomatoes are soft and the okra is tender, 5-7 minutes.

California Medley

6 Portions • 40 Calories, 2 grams of Fat

8 ounces	peeled baby carrots
8 ounces	cauliflower florettes
8 ounces	broccoli florettes
1 tbsp	unsalted butter, melted
1/2 tsp	kosher salt
1/8 tsp	black pepper

Fit a steamer basket into the bottom of a 4-5 quart pot. Add water until it reaches the base of the basket. Cover the steamer and bring to a boil over high heat. When the water is boiling, add the carrots and cover, steaming for 5 minutes. After 5 minutes, add the cauliflower and after a second 5 minutes, the broccoli. When all the vegetables are tender, 5-7 minutes after the broccoli is added, remove them from the steamer. Toss with butter, salt and pepper.

Garlic Broccoli

6 Portions • 45 Calories, 1.5 grams of Fat

1 1/2 lbs	broccoli florettes
1 1/2 tsps	olive oil
2 cloves	garlic, minced
1/2 tsp	kosher salt
1/2 tsp	granulated sugar
1/4 tsp	crushed red pepper flakes

Bring a large pot of water to a boil and cook the broccoli for 2 minutes. Drain well and rinse with cold water to stop the broccoli from cooking further. Place the remaining ingredients in a cold, nonstick skillet. With the burner on medium high heat, sauté the pepper, garlic, salt and sugar until the garlic is golden brown and fragrant. Add the broccoli to the pan and toss to re-warm and coat with the garlic.

Buttered Sugar Snap Peas

6 Portions • 85 Calories, 2.5 grams of Fat

1 1/2 lbs	sugar snap peas, washed and trimmed
1 tbsp	unsalted butter
1/2 tsp	kosher salt
	pinch black pepper

Bring a large pot of water to a boil. Boil the peas for 4-5 minutes, until tender. Drain well. Stir in the butter and season with salt and pepper.

Sugar Snap Pea and Pecorino Salad

6 Portions • 110 Calories, 4 grams of Fat

1 1/2 lbs	sugar snap peas, cleaned and trimmed
1 tbsp	olive oil
1 ounce	grated pecorino cheese
1/2 tbsp	red wine vinegar
1/2 tsp	dried oregano
1/8 tsp	dried thyme
1/2 tsp	kosher salt
	pinch black pepper

Bring a large pot of water to a boil. Boil the peas for 3-4 minutes, until tender, but still crisp. Drain and immediately rinse with cold water. Chill. In a large bowl combine olive oil, red wine vinegar, oregano, thyme, salt and pepper. Add grated pecorino cheese, then toss peas with the dressing. Chill for at least 15 minutes more before serving.

Roasted Seaphire (Sea Asparagus)

6 Portions • 40 Calories, 0 grams of Fat

24 ounces	seaphire
	non-stick cooking spray
	kosher salt
	ground black pepper

Preheat oven to 400 degrees. Wash seaphire and trim the stems and discard. Arrange in a single layer on foil lined baking sheets. Coat the seaphire evenly with cooking spray. Roast 5-7 minutes, depending on the thickness of the spears. Remove from the oven and season with salt and pepper.

Cinnamon Apples

6 Portions • 120 Calories, 2 grams of Fat

4 cups	frozen sliced apples, without sugar
1 tbsp	unsalted butter
1/3 cup	packed brown sugar
1 tsp	ground cinnamon
1/4 tsp	kosher salt

Preheat oven to 325 degrees. Melt the butter. Combine apples with the butter, brown sugar and cinnamon. Place covered in the oven for 45 minutes. Then, uncover and bake 15-20 minutes more, until most of the liquid has evaporated and a syrup has formed around the apples.

Buttered Cauliflower

6 Portions • 175 Calories, 3.5 grams of Fat

24 ounces	cauliflower florettes
1 tbsp	butter
	kosher salt
	black pepper

Place steamer basket in the bottom of a large pot with a cover. Fill the base with water, cover and bring the water to a boil. Add the cauliflower, cover and allow to steam 10-12 minutes, until tender crisp. Remove from steamer, toss with butter and season with salt and pepper.

Snack Guide

Dried Fruit

1 ounce dried apples	75 Calories, 0 grams of Fat
1 ounce dried apricots	65 Calories, 0 grams of Fat
1 ounce sweetened, dried cranberries	95 Calories, 0 grams of Fat
1 ounce dried currants	80 Calories, 0 grams of Fat
1 ounce dried dates	80 Calories, 0 grams of Fat
1 ounce dried fig pieces	70 Calories, 0 grams of Fat
1 ounce dried peaches	60 Calories, 0 grams of Fat
1 ounce dried pears	75 Calories, 0 grams of Fat
1 ounce dried pineapple pieces	80 Calories, 0 grams of Fat
1 ounce prunes with pits	60 Calories, 0 grams of Fat
1 ounce raisins	90 Calories, 0 grams of Fat
1/2 cup applesauce, sweetened	90 Calories, 0 grams of Fat
1/2 cup sugarfree, fruit gelatin	10 Calories, 0 grams of Fat

Fresh Fruit

Apple, medium (5.5 ounce)	90 Calories, 0 grams of Fat
Banana, medium (8 ounce)	80 Calories, 0 grams of Fat
Blueberries/Blackberries (1/2 cup)	40 Calories, 0 grams of Fat
Cantaloupe (1 cup)	55 Calories, 0 grams of Fat
Cherries (8 sweet)	40 Calories, 0 grams of Fat
Grapefruit 1/2, (10 ounces)	55 Calories, 0 grams of Fat
Grapes (1 cup)	100 Calories, 0 grams of Fat
Honeydew melon (1 cup)	60 Calories, 0 grams of Fat
Kiwifruit, medium (3 ounce)	45 Calories, 0 grams of Fat
Nectarine, medium (4 ounce)	50 Calories, 0 grams of Fat
Orange, medium (7 ounce)	70 Calories, 0 grams of Fat
Peach, medium (4 ounce)	35 Calories, 0 grams of Fat
Pear, medium (6 ounce)	90 Calories, 0 grams of Fat
Pineapple (1 cup)	75 Calories, 0 grams of Fat
Plum, medium (3 ounce)	45 Calories, 0 grams of Fat
Raspberries (1/2 cup)	30 Calories, 0 grams of Fat

Eucalorics

Snack Guide

Strawberries (1 cup) ....45 Calories, 0 grams of Fat

Tangerine, medium (4 ounce)..................................50 Calories, 0 grams of Fat

Watermelon (1 cup) ....50 Calories, 0 grams of Fat

Nuts

1 ounce almonds ....170 Calories, 15 grams of Fat

1 ounce cashews ....165 Calories, 14 grams of Fat

1 ounce peanuts ....120 Calories, 10 grams of Fat

1 ounce pecans ....190 Calories, 19 grams of Fat

1 ounce walnuts ....175 Calories, 16 grams of Fat

1 ounce avg. mixed nuts ....175 Calories, 13 grams of Fat

1 ounce sunflower seeds ....160 Calories, 14 grams of Fat

1 tablespoon peanut butter ....105 Calories, 8.5 grams of Fat

Dairy

8 ounces nonfat fruit yogurt ....120 Calories, 0 grams of Fat

1/2 cup lowfat (1%) cottage cheese ....80 Calories, 1 gram of Fat

1 ounce cheddar cheese..110 Calories, 9 grams of Fat

1 ounce string cheese ....80 Calories, 5 grams of Fat

1 ounce swiss cheese ....110 Calories, 9 grams of Fat

1/2 cup nonfat pudding, choc./vanilla ....100 Calories, 0 grams of Fat

1/2 cup fruit sherbet..120 Calories, 2 grams of Fat

1/2 cup fruit sorbet..120 Calories, 0 grams of Fat

Fat free fudgesicle ....60 Calories, 0 grams of Fat

Orange creamsicle...110 Calories, 3 grams of Fat

1/2 cup soft serve low fat frozen yogurt ....120 Calories, 2.5 grams of Fat

1/2 cup soft serve nonfat frozen yogurt ....100 Calories, 0 grams of Fat

Salty Snacks

1 ounce WOW™, Tostitos, chips ....90 Calories, 0 grams of Fat

1 ounce WOW™, Doritos, chips ....90 Calories, 0 grams of Fat

1 ounce WOW™, Potato chips, all varieties.............75 Calories, 0 grams of Fat

Snack Guide

1 ounce pretzels ....110 Calories, 2 grams of Fat

1 ounce animal crackers ....130 Calories, 2 grams of Fat

55 plain goldfish crackers ....140 Calories, 6 grams of Fat

8 graham crackers ....120 Calories, 2 grams of Fat

Granola/cereal bars, avg. ....130 Calories, 3 grams of Fat

1 cup light, microwave popcorn................................25 Calories, 1 gram of Fat

Sweets

2 Chips Ahoy! cookies ....160 Calories, 8 grams of Fat

2 Fig Newtons ....220 Calories, 5 grams of Fat

5 Ginger Snaps ....150 Calories, 6 grams of Fat

1 Nutty Bar (2 ounce) ....155 Calories, 9 grams of Fat

1 Oatmeal Creme Pie ....170 Calories, 7 grams of Fat

3 Oreo cookies ....160 Calories, 7 grams of Fat

2 Soft Batch cookies (.5 ounce) ....160 Calories, 7 grams of Fat

10 vanilla wafers ....150 Calories, 5 grams of Fat

2 Vienna fingers ....140 Calories, 6 grams of Fat

Coldstone Creamery®

4 ounces chocolate ice cream ....240 Calories, 14 grams of Fat

4 ounces Italian sorbet ....110 Calories, 0 grams of Fat

4 ounces sweet cream ice cream ....260 Calories, 16 grams of Fat

4 ounces yogurt ....140 Calories, 0 grams of Fat

McDonald's®

Low fat vanilla ice cream cone ....150 Calories, 4.5 grams of Fat

Mrs. Fields Cookies®

Butter cookie ....220 Calories, 10 grams of Fat

Butter toffee ....220 Calories, 10 grams of Fat

Chewy fudge ....300 Calories, 12 grams of Fat

Cinnamon sugar ....300 Calories, 12 grams of Fat

Eucalorics

Snack Guide

Coconut macadamia ....280 Calories, 13 grams of Fat
Debra's special...280 Calories, 12 grams of Fat
Milk chocolate ....230 Calories, 11 grams of Fat
Milk chocolate with walnuts/macadamia nuts ....320 Calories, 18 grams of Fat
Milk chocolate chip ....280 Calories, 13 grams of Fat
Oatmeal chocolate chip ....280 Calories, 13 grams of Fat
Oatmeal raisin ....180 Calories, 7 grams of Fat
Peanut butter ....310 Calories, 16 grams of Fat
Peanut butter milk chocolate ....300 Calories, 17 grams of Fat
Pumpkin harvest..200 Calories, 10 grams of Fat
Semi-sweet chocolate ....280 Calories, 14 grams of Fat
Semi-sweet chocolate with walnuts/macadamia nuts..............310 Calories, 16 grams of Fat
Triple chocolate ....220 Calories, 10 grams of Fat
White chunk macadamia ....310 Calories, 17 grams of Fat

Starbuck's® (all numbers based on Grande, 16 fluid ounces)
Caffe latté with whole milk ....270 Calories, 14 grams of Fat
Caffe latté with 2% milk ....220 Calories, 7 grams of Fat
Caffe latté with skim milk ....160 Calories, 1 gram of Fat
Cappuccino with whole milk ....180 Calories, 9 grams of Fat
Cappuccino with 2% milk ....140 Calories, 5 grams of Fat
Cappuccino with skim milk ....110 Calories, 0 grams of Fat
Chai tea latté with whole milk ....320 Calories, 13 grams of Fat
Chai tea latté with Skim milk ....210 Calories, .5 grams of Fat
Coffee frappuccino ....270 Calories, 3.5 grams of Fat
Tazo Berry ....210 Calories, 0 grams of Fat
Tazo Berry & Cream ....600 Calories, 23 grams of Fat

Fast Food Options

Atlanta Bread Company®

French Roll ....180 Calories, .5 gram of Fat

Sourdough Roll ....190 Calories, 0 grams of Fat

Cup of soup:

Baked Potato ....210 Calories, 13 grams of Fat

Barley and Sage ....80 Calories, 1 gram of Fat

Black Bean with Ham...200 Calories. 7 grams of Fat

Black Bean & Rice ....110 Calories, 3 grams of Fat

Chicken Chili...220 Calories, 6 grams of Fat

Chicken Gumbo...110 Calories, 3 grams of Fat

Chicken 'n Dumpling..240 Calories, 13 grams of Fat

Chicken Noodle ....110 Calories, 4 grams of Fat

Chicken Tortilla ....140 Calories, 7 grams of Fat

Chili w. Beans..280 Calories, 11 grams of Fat

Clam Chowder ....270 Calories, 16 grams of Fat

Country Bean ....140 Calories, 4.5 grams of Fat

Cream of Broccoli..150 Calories, 9 grams of Fat

French Onion...60 Calories, 2 grams of Fat

Garden Vegetable...80 Calories, 1 gram of Fat

Italian Style Wedding ....120 Calories, 3 grams of Fat

Lentil & Roasted Garlic..200 Calories, 2.5 grams of Fat

Mushroom ....80 Calories, 1 gram of Fat

Pasta Fagioli ....160 Calories, 6 grams of Fat

Seven Bean w. Ham ....240 Calories, 12 grams of Fat

Southwest Chicken ....180 Calories, 9 grams of Fat

Szechuan Hot & Sour ....80 Calories, 2 grams of Fat

Tomato Florentine ....120 Calories, 3 grams of Fat

Tomato, Fennel & Dill..100 Calories, 7 grams of Fat

Vegetable Chili ....180 Calories, 3.5 grams of Fat

Wisconsin Cheese..210 Calories, 11 grams of Fat

Back Yard Burgers®

Cup Chili & Garden Salad, dressing on the side ....295 Calories, 12 grams of Fat

Bar-B-Que Chicken Sandwich ....290 Calories, 7 grams of Fat

Eucalorics

Fast Food Options

Blackened Chicken Sandwich .... 320 Calories, 11 grams of Fat

Hawaiian Chicken Sandwich .... 310 Calories, 11 grams of Fat

Honey Mustard Chicken Sandwich .... 380 Calories, 8.5 grams Fat

Lemon Butter Chicken Sandwich .... 300 Calories, 11 grams of Fat

Mexicali Chicken Sandwich .... 350 Calories, 9 grams of Fat

Miz Grazi's Chicken Sandwich .... 290 Calories, 4 grams of Fat

Savory Chicken Sandwich .... 270 Calories, 4 grams of Fat

Great Little Burger® .... 280 Calories, 15 grams of Fat

Gardenburger ® .... 330 Calories, 5.5 grams Fat

Blimpie®

6" subs on white, with lettuce, tomato, & onion

Blimpie Best .... 410 Calories, 13 grams of Fat

Club Sub .... 370 Calories, 10 grams of Fat

Ham & Swiss .... 410 Calories, 14 grams of Fat

Roast Beef .... 390 Calories, 7 grams of Fat

Turkey Sub .... 330 Calories, 6 grams of Fat

Grilled Chicken .... 400 Calories, 9 grams of Fat

Mexi Max .... 395 Calories, 4.5 grams of Fat

Roast Turkey Cordon Bleu .... 430 Calories, 14 grams of Fat

Veggie Max .... 405 Calories, 7 grams of Fat

Burger King®

Whopper JR, Sandwich®, no Mayonnaise .... 310 Calories, 13 grams of Fat

Whopper JR, w/ Cheese®, no Mayonnaise .... 360 Calories, 19 grams of Fat

BK Veggie™ Burger .... 360 Calories, 10 grams of Fat

Chicken Whopper Jr, no Mayonnaise .... 270 Calories, 6 grams of Fat

Chick-Fil-A®

Chargrilled Chicken Sandwich Deluxe .... 280 Calories, 7 grams of Fat

Chargrilled Chicken Sandwich, no butter .... 240 Calories, 3.5 grams Fat

Chargrilled Chicken Garden Salad, dressing on the side .... 180 Calories, 6 grams of Fat

Chicken Caesar Salad, dressing on the side .... 240 Calories, 10 grams of Fat

Fast Food Options

Fazoli's® Italian Food

Minestrone Soup & buttered breadstick ....260 Calories, 7 grams of Fat

Minestrone Soup & dry bread stick ....210 Calories, 2 grams of Fat

Small Spaghetti with Marinara ....420 Calories, 6 grams of Fat

Small Spaghetti with Meat Sauce ....450 Calories, 8 grams of Fat

Double Slice Cheese Pizza ....460 Calories, 15 grams of Fat

Jimmy John's®

Sandwiches on French Bread, no mayonnaise

Big John ....330 Calories, 3 grams of Fat

Bootlegger Club..435 Calories, 3.5 grams of Fat

Bootlegger Club w. Cheese...485 Calories, 8 grams of Fat

Ham & Cheese..405 Calories, 10 grams of Fat

Roast Beef...365 Calories, 3 grams of Fat

The Pepe w. Cheese ....370 Calories, 10 grams of Fat

Turkey Tom ....310 Calories, 1 gram of Fat

Turkey Tom with Cheese ....425 Calories, 8 grams of Fat

McDonald's®

Hamburger..280 Calories, 10 grams of Fat

Cheeseburger ....330 Calories, 14 grams of Fat

Chicken McGrill®, no mayonnaise ....300 Calories, 6 grams of Fat

Fruit & Yogurt Parfait...380 Calories, 5 grams of Fat

Fruit & Yogurt Parfait w/out Granola.....................................280 Calories, 4 grams of Fat

Grilled Bacon Chicken Ranch Salad, no dressing ....250 Calories, 10 grams of Fat

Grilled Chicken Caesar Salad, no dressing ....200 Calories, 6 grams of Fat

Grilled Chicken California Cobb Salad, no dressing...............270 Calories, 11 grams of Fat

Panera Bread®

French roll ....140 Calories, 1 gram of Fat

Sourdough roll ....160 Calories, 0 grams of Fat

Cup of Soup

Baked Potato ....240 Calories, 15 grams of Fat

Beef & 3 Bean Chili..250 Calories, 9 grams of Fat

Eucalorics

Fast Food Options

Broccoli Cheddar	220 Calories, 17 grams of Fat
Chicken Noodle	110 Calories, 2.5 grams of Fat
Cream of Chicken & Wild Rice	210 Calories, 13 grams of Fat
Fire Roasted Vegetable Bisque	180 Calories, 11 grams of Fat
Forest Mushroom	140 Calories, 8 grams of Fat
Fresh Onion	80 Calories, 3 grams of Fat
Mesa Vegetable & Bean	100 Calories, .5 grams of Fat
Potato Cream Cheese	190 Calories, 10 grams of Fat
Savory Vegetable Bean	120 Calories, 2 grams of Fat
Sirloin Beef	210 Calories, 10 grams of Fat
Vegetarian Black Bean	180 Calories, .5 grams of Fat
Vegetarian Lentil Soup	120 Calories, 2 grams of Fat
Vegetarian Vegetable Gumbo	110 Calories, 3 grams of Fat
White Chicken Chili	180 Calories, 6 grams of Fat

Sonic Drive-In®

Jr. Burger	355 Calories, 21 grams of Fat
Grilled Cheese	280 Calories, 12 grams of Fat
Grilled Chicken Sandwich	345 Calories, 13 grams of Fat
Grilled Chicken Wrap, w/out dressing	395 Calories, 12 grams of Fat

Subway®

6" Sub on Italian, with lettuce, tomato, onion, green pepper, pickles and olives

Ham	290 Calories, 5 grams of Fat
Roast Beef	290 Calories, 5 grams of Fat
Roasted Chicken Breast	320 Calories, 5 grams of Fat
SUBWAY Club®	320 Calories, 6 grams of Fat
Turkey Breast	280 Calories, 4.5 grams of Fat
Turkey Breast & Ham	290 Calories, 5 grams of Fat
Veggie Delight,	230 Calories, 3 grams of Fat

Taco Bell®

Bean Burrito	370 Calories, 12 grams of Fat
Beef Taco, regular	210 Calories, 12 grams of Fat

Fast Food

Fast Food Options

Beef Taco, supreme ....260 Calories, 16 grams of Fat
Soft Beef Taco...210 Calories, 10 grams of Fat
Soft Chicken Taco ....190 Calories, 7 grams of Fat
Gordita Baja™ Beef..360 Calories, 21 grams of Fat
Gordita Baja™ Chicken or Steak..340 Calories, 18 grams of Fat
Gordita Supreme® Beef or Steak ....300 Calories, 14 grams of Fat
Gordita Supreme® Chicken..300 Calories, 13 grams of Fat
Pintos 'n Cheese ....180 Calories, 8 grams of Fat
Mexican Rice ....190 Calories, 9 grams of Fat
Tostada ....250 Calories, 12 grams of Fat
Meximelt®...290 Calories, 15 grams of Fat
Taco Salad w. Salsa w/out shell ....400 Calories, 22 grams of Fat

Wendy's®

Chicken BLT Salad, no dressing ....310 Calories, 16 grams of Fat
Mandarin Chicken Salad™, no dressing, nuts, or noodles ....150 Calories, 1.5 grams of Fat
Taco Supreme Salad, no chips or sour cream ....390 Calories, 17 grams of Fat
Grilled Chicken Sandwich ....300 Calories, 7 grams of Fat
Jr. Hamburger ....270 Calories, 9 grams of Fat
Jr. Cheeseburger ....310 Calories, 12 grams of Fat

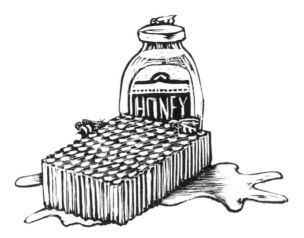

Index

Recipe Index

Recipe Index

Recipe Index

Recipe Index